HEAL THE CHILDREN

How Schools Promote Disease
How Parents Can Take Action

Angela K. Griffiths DC
Kelson H. Griffiths

This publication contains the opinions and ideas of the authors. It is intended to provide helpful and informative material on the subjects addressed in the publication. It is sold with the understanding that the authors and publisher are not engaged in rendering medical, health, nutritional, psychological, or any other kind of personal professional services in the book. If the reader requires personal medical attention, health, nutritional, or other assistance or advice, a competent professional should be consulted.

The authors and publisher specifically disclaim all responsibility for any liability, loss, or risk, personal or otherwise, that is incurred as a consequence, directly or indirectly, of the use and application of any of the contents of this book.

Printed in the United States of America.

Library of Congress Cataloging in Publication Data

Griffiths, Angela, 2015 –
Heal the children : how schools promote disease, how parents can take action / Angela Griffiths, Kelson Griffiths

For ordering information, visit: www.angelagriffithsdc/healthechildren.

Cover photo by Crystal Palmer Bull.

ISBN-13: 978-0692398012
ISBN-10: 0692398015

For

all parents who truly just want the best for their children and are confused by all the conflicting information

For

my parents who encouraged me to keep asking the difficult questions

For

my children, parents and siblings who are on this quest of learning, growing and teaching with me.

Thank you to so many friends and family who helped make this book possible: Kim Windsor, Jane Knowles, Anjanette Fennell, Jane Hansen, and Aubrey Schreck for research or editing support.

TABLE OF CONTENTS

INTRODUCTION

How did it come to be that we lost our common sense about food? I say we, because I too have fallen down the rabbit hole, confused about how I should eat to build muscle, lose fat, improve memory and stay healthy. I am of the generation that grew up with the Dairy Industry, Meat Industry, Pharmaceutical Industry, Diet Industry, Candy Industry, and every other "industry" marketing to us from cradle to grave. Our children have learned to sing advertising jingles for processed foods before they even enter school.

The mass advertising of unhealthy food and confusing health messages, the industrialization of farming and the creation of Frankenstein-like-foods has all happened in my generation. Isn't it interesting to note that in that same time period rates of ADHD, obesity, diabetes, cancers, heart disease, numerous autoimmune diseases, and metabolic syndrome have also skyrocketed (and are starting at younger and younger ages)? It's not a coincidence. The fox has been not only allowed in the hen house, the fox *lives* in the hen house now.

> *"More people are realizing there are myriad chemicals in conventionally produced food," says Craig Minowa, environmental scientist with the Organic Consumers Association, a nonprofit advocacy group. Although each has passed its own safety review, Minowa points out that "Most of the studies on safety are done or supported by the companies themselves."*

Studies have shown that how we eat in our childhood sets the foundation for our adult and lifetime health. Some diseases, previously only seen in adulthood, are becoming more prevalent in childhood (e.g. obesity and Type 2 diabetes). Other diseases can take decades to develop, but we are now seeing them in 20- and 30-year-olds instead of 50- and 60-year-olds (e.g. cancers, metabolic syndrome, hypertension and even heart disease). In fact, this is the

1

first generation of children that are not expected to outlive their parents. Their foundation has been constructed of quick sand.

My youngest child, since birth, has had many digestive issues, was always bloated, puffy and gassy. He has had severe "seasonal allergies" since about the age of 5. Of my three children, he caught the most colds and stayed sick longer. During middle school he came down with a cold or flu, like many children do. His fever quickly advanced to 103 degrees and I got him to a doctor (since it was a Friday preceding a 3-day weekend). Because most doctors dismiss a fever that has only been around for 24-36 hours, he was sent home with no treatment. On Sunday the fever and symptoms had not subsided and I was truly concerned. I took him to an urgent care center where they immediately ordered an x-ray. He was diagnosed with an aggressive case of pneumonia, "One of the worst [they had] ever seen in a child that walked themselves in to the clinic." His immune system had been severely compromised.

At the age of 13, conscientious of his new acne-covered face and long-time bloated belly, my son asked if going gluten- and dairy-free might make a difference. Despite not accepting the milk offered at lunch, my son was still offered and regularly consumed other forms of dairy. My response to his inquiry, "It certainly couldn't make it worse." Together we embarked on an elimination diet that confirmed his sensitivities to both gluten and dairy. He immediately lost weight, his "puffy belly" and almost all digestive issues. He also strengthened his immune system and is now rarely affected by flus and/or colds suffered by his peers. His seasonal allergies have improved greatly. Occasionally sugar intake fuels more acne. But, as a teen, he is not completely free from the culture in which he lives. Sugar, sugar everywhere!

All of my children attended public schools and I had to fight to try to protect their health and nutrition. Each of my children showed dairy sensitivities from their first exposure. Not a true anaphylactic allergy, but a sensitivity nonetheless: increasing mucous production, ear infections, etc. Doctors said they would grow out of it. Clearly, they did not. The Dairy Industry (National Dairy Council) underwrites portions of the school breakfast and school lunch programs in public schools. Students are always offered milk and milk alone (or sometimes tap water) *unless* they have a documented allergy. The Dairy Council also creates and offers, free of charge, "health" curriculum to schools. The misleading content contained in these curricula will be discussed further in a later chapter.

It was the quest and struggles of my youngest son to maintain his newfound healthy lifestyle while attending public schools that became the inspiration of this book. Together, we hope that the information contained herein touches a core for you, saves you from going through what we have had to go through, encourages you to educate your own children about nutrition, and provides a blueprint for how to help change the current system so that more kids can thrive.

PART I

DANGEROUS FOODS COMMONLY FOUND ON SCHOOL CAMPUSES

The common thread among all chronic disease is inflammation. Low levels of cellular irritation happen for years prior to a diagnosis of a disease. Obesity is inflammation of adipose tissue (or fat cells).[i] Diabetes is inflammation of the pancreas.[ii,iii] Heart disease is inflammation of blood vessels.[iv] Cancer is inflammation of the immune system.[v] Alzheimer's is inflammation of the brain. I think you get the picture.

Causes of Cellular Inflammation:[vi]

1. **Increased Omega 6 Consumption**—increasing hormones that cause inflammation
2. **Increased Refined Carbohydrate Consumption**—flours, sugars, "processed" food causing blood sugar instability and insulin responses
3. **Decreased Omega 3 Consumption**—causing an Omega 6 to Omega 3 imbalance, leading to a loss in the ability to protect against inflammation
4. **Decreased Polyphenol Consumption**—antioxidants; found in plants; decreasing consumption causes a loss in the ability to protect against chronic diseases and cancer

5. **Low Fiber Intake**—fiber is primarily found in raw vegetables and fruits as well as whole, unprocessed, grains; dietary fiber is protective against inflammation[vii]

How and why are foods found on school campuses causing and contributing to inflammation in children? Our children are basically eating fast food on school campuses: high amounts of refined carbohydrates (cereals, pancakes, cinnamon rolls, breads, pastas, pizza crust), high amounts of Omega 6 fats (processed grains and vegetable oils) accompanied by a high amount of saturated fats (animal foods—milk, cheese, meat), with a deficiency of Omega 3 fats (flax seeds, walnuts, sardines, salmon, soybeans, shrimp, Brussel sprouts, cauliflower and winter squash) and polyphenols (fruits, vegetables, legumes, nuts and seeds, dark chocolate, tea and many seasonings).

Processed and Frankenstein-like foods that we consume are killing us. The foods that we will look at in this section have all been shown to encourage disease promotion in both the short and the long term. About 90 percent of the money Americans spend on food is spent on processed foods.[viii] This includes restaurant foods (e.g. food away from home, including school cafeterias) and processed grocery foods that require little or no preparation time before consuming. In order to take care of your (and your children's) health, you must understand how food was grown, what is in it and how it can either harm or heal your health.

The Food and Nutrition Service (FNS) of the United States Department of Agriculture (USDA) is responsible for the policies behind the food that is allowed on school campuses. At its inception, the USDA had the dual responsibility of protecting the interests of citizens and farmers. But today there are fewer and fewer small family farms, as they have been gradually and almost completely taken over by factory farms (the Farming Industry).

The USDA has the responsibility for two seemingly competitive interests: the health of citizens (including our children) and the profit and survival of the Farming Industry.

Farm subsidies used to help Mom-and-Pop-Farmers through rough seasons, and the backbone of our nation's food supply used to be small family farms, which protected their land, took pride over the quality of their food and rotated crops to keep pests under control. Now our food supply is being controlled by corporations whose primary goal is profit. The Farming Industry has seemingly no respect for the land, the quality of the food grown on it, or the sustainability of our ecosystem based on their farming practices. And they are backed by large chemical companies who have essentially changed the face of farming to make a profit through pesticides and genetically modified crops.

In fact, most of the grain grown in North America today is not for human consumption, but for livestock and almost *all of it* is treated with, or genetically modified to include, pesticides, herbicides and/or insecticides.

Our tax dollars (through the Farm Bill) are now used to over-produce food that is of poor quality, chemically contaminated and is putting our health at risk (and which is shipped into our schools for consumption!).

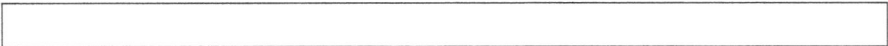

According to Jeff Gillman, PhD, associate professor of horticulture at the University of Minnesota and author of *The Truth About Organic Gardening*, "Modern production of foods incorporates a wide range of synthetic chemicals." And continues, "Many of these chemicals have the potential to be very damaging to humans if they are exposed to high concentrations, or to low concentrations over an extended period of time."

2010 Dietary Guidelines for Americans

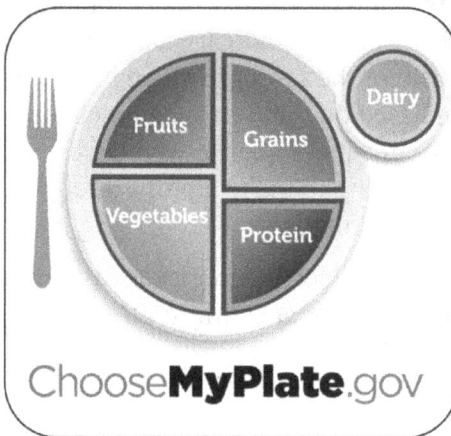

In the name of keeping us healthy, the USDA is tasked with creating *Dietary Guidelines for Americans*. The guidelines are reviewed every five years and have been criticized as not accurately representing scientific information about optimal nutrition, and as being overly influenced by dairy, agricultural and other industries.

School curricula and public education campaigns are developed based on these guidelines, with many still reflecting the views of guidelines that were thrown out ten years ago (the *Food Pyramid* and *MyPyramid)*. The Dairy Industry (National Dairy Council) has had a strong hand through lobbying and still retains their own "spot" on the current revision of the guidelines (2010), despite the fact that milk is simply another source of protein and carbohydrate and has been tied to health and digestive issues in many people. There remain concerns with the present guidelines that will hopefully be dealt with and result in revisions upon the next review in 2015.

Two problematic themes of nutrition throughout history:

1) Investigate nutrients and nutrient events in isolation

By isolating nutrients, food companies can focus on one particular nutrient and "add" what they think you might need or what might be missing from their processed food-like-product. Following the same thinking, vitamin companies promote that you can take their pill to get what you need (rather than eating it from whole food). While nutrients have been somewhat broken up in this section to highlight and show you some of the problems of them individually, we absolutely must remember that natural food in history did not contain only one ingredient—ever!

2) Focus on protein

Protein is not a "super food," it is not the most important nutrient that we take on *and* it is not just available from animal sources (meat, milk, fish, etc.). In fact, many would say that there *is* an upper limit to how much protein we should take in, as it does promote growth (thus body builders tend to eat it, almost in isolation of all other nutrients). But it also has a downside (as does anything eaten to excess). Protein has been shown in research to not only increase the growth of muscles; it also increases the growth of tumor cells (through IGF-1 activity).[ix] More is not always better.

Broccoli can be used as a great example to make both of these points. Broccoli does not just contain one nutrient. There is no supplement out there that you can take to obtain all of the benefits from eating the whole plant called broccoli. As far as micronutrients go, it contains vitamins A, C, D, E, K, B1 (Thiamin), B2 (Riboflavin), B3 (Niacin), B6, B9 (folate), B12, Pantothenic Acid, Choline and Betaine. Yes, in case you got lost, we are *still* talking about the ingredients in plain ol' broccoli. It contains antioxidants and phytonutrients known to prevent cancer and other diseases. It contains fiber which helps bind to and eliminate toxins and prevent colon and bowel cancers. It also contains carbohydrates, fats *and proteins!* You heard (read) me correctly. Broccoli contains three grams of protein per serving and because of its high fiber content, it helps you to feel more "satiated" (or content, full, happy belly!).

So what have the alphabet soup of government agencies (USDA, FDA, EPA and others) allowed and promoted to be present in our children's food at school and on many of our plates at home? I hope you read on to find out!

---

[i] Gregor MF and Hotamisligil GS. Inflammatory mechanisms in obesity. Annu Rev Immunol. 2011;29:415-45. http://www.ncbi.nlm.nih.gov/pubmed/21219177; available August 13, 2014.

[ii] Cosentino F and Egidy Assenza G. Diabetes and Inflammation. Herz Dec 2004;29(8):749-759.

[iii] Dandona P et al. Metabolic Syndrome: A Comprehensive Perspective Based on Interactions Between Obesity, Diabetes, and Inflammation. http://www.yorktest-tr.com/pdf/18-Metabolic-Syndrome-A-Comprehensive-Perspective-Based-on-Interactions-Between-Obesity-Diabetes-and-Inflammation.pdf; available August 13, 2014.

[iv] Pearson T et al. AHA/CDC Scientific Statement: Markers of Inflammation and Cardiovascular Disease. http://circ.ahajournals.org/content/107/3/499.full; available August 8, 2014.

[v] Mantovani A et al. Review Article Cancer-related inflammation. Nature 454, 436-444 (24 July 2008); http://www.nature.com/nature/journal/v454/n7203/full/nature07205.html; available August 13, 2014.

[vi] Sears, Barry. Enter The Zone—A Dietary Roadmap. HarperCollins, 1995.

[vii] Association between dietary fiber and serum C-Reactive protein: http://ajcn.nutrition.org/content/83/4/760.full

[viii] Eric Schlosser, Fast Food Nation, 2012, Penguin Books: http://jhampton.pbworks.com/w/file/fetch/51769044/Fast%20Food%20Nation.pdf.

[ix] Youngman LD, and Campbell TC. "Inhibition of aflatoxin B1-induced gamma-glutamyl transpeptidase positive (GGT+) hepatic preneoplastic foci and tumors by low protein diets: evidence that altered GGT+ foci indicate neoplastic potential." Carciogenesis 13(1992):1609-1613.

CHAPTER 1

SUGAR

Of all possible dietary culprits, sugar, especially processed fructose, wins top billing as the "greatest destroyer of health."[x] Research shows that sugar consumption has increased annually since 1982. In 2000, each American consumed an average of 152 pounds (or roughly 68,946 grams) of sugar. That's 2/5 of a pound—52 teaspoons, or 208 grams—of added sugars per person per day.[xi] Sources of this sugar commonly include cane sugar, beet sugar, corn syrup and corn sugar. The American Heart Association recommends no more than 11 cubes of sugar (or roughly 100 calories) for women per day and 16.5 cubes (or roughly 150 calories) for men per day.

How Much Sugar Are You Consuming?

Food	Sugar grams	Cubes	Calories	% Daily Recommendation	
				Men	Women
Candy Bar	24g	10	96	64%	96%
8.3 oz. can of energy drink	27g	12	108	72%	108%
Pint of vanilla ice cream	84g	36.5	336	224%	336%
Liter of soda	124g	54	496	331%	496%
2 pancakes with ¼ c. syrup	50g	22	200	133%	200%
Cookie	18g	8	72	48%	72%

You can see by reading this chart how easily people are exceeding recommended levels of sugar consumption.

A high level of sugar consumption has clear health consequences. One recent study, looking at the relationships between added sugar and heart disease found that:

- Most adults (just over 71 percent) get 10 percent or more of their daily calories from added sugar.

- Approximately 10 percent of American adults got 25 percent or more of their daily calories from added sugar in 2005-2010.

- The most common sources of added sugar are sugar-sweetened beverages, grain-based desserts, fruit drinks, dairy desserts, and candy.

- Those who consume 21 percent or more of their daily calories in the form of sugar are *twice* as likely to die from heart disease as compared to those who get seven percent or less of their daily calories from added sugar.[xii]

Sugar-sweetened beverages dramatically increase your risk of metabolic syndrome, Type 2 diabetes, heart disease and mortality.[xiii] One study showed that it only took two weeks for subjects consuming high-fructose corn syrup to have increased blood levels of LDL cholesterol and other risk factors for cardiovascular disease.[xiv] Diet sodas or artificially sweetened foods and beverages are no better, as research reveals that they appear to do even *more* harm than refined sugar or high fructose corn syrup, causing even *greater* weight gain.[xv]

Sugar has been shown to induce cancer. When we eat or drink sugar, it causes a spike in the hormone insulin, which can serve as a catalyst to fuel certain types of cancers, including breast and colon. Tumors with insulin receptors can be stimulated by a high intake of glucose from the blood stream the sugar actually "feeds" the cancer growth.[xvi]

Sugar is addictive, activating the brain similar to drugs like cocaine. Dopamine, a chemical to stimulate the brain's pleasure center, is released with the intake of sugar, just as it would with drugs or alcohol. People who frequently consume sweetened food and beverages may build up a tolerance, much like drug users do. The more you eat, the less you feel the reward. The result: you eat more and more to achieve the same feeling.[xvii]

Sugar causes you to be unable to think clearly due to impaired brain cell signaling (decreased sensitivity due to chronic high blood glucose levels). Understanding sugar's link to diseases and its effect on the brain, there should be an absolute limit, combined limit, of how much sugar kids consume across all school environments (cafeteria, snack bars, vending machines, classroom incentives and parties, etc.). Parents, knowing these limits, would have a better ability to monitor and limit further sugar intake beyond school hours in order to protect their child's health.

At present, the USDA has no limit on the amount of sugar that can be served in school meals.

Clearly the USDA is lagging and has yet to create or implement policies with regard to school nutrition subsequent to the vast amount of research regarding sugar and high fructose corn syrup. According to a *Facebook* post on August 20, 2014, one absolutely frustrated mom posts:

> *I am so disgusted! My kids met their teachers today. (They start school tomorrow.) As we were walking in, a couple of the lunch ladies were wheeling in*

enormous boxes and dropping them off inside each classroom. The boxes were filled with Trix, Lucky Charms, and Cinnamon Toast Crunch cereals!! Our school provides free breakfast for all children (Pre-K through 4th grade), and this is the offering along with Pop-Tarts, French toast sticks, and pancakes! I was very clear with both my kids' teachers that I will make sure they have breakfast before school every morning. If they are hungry, they can have a piece of fruit in the classroom. It's just so hard to understand how someone could think this is perfectly acceptable to order and serve to kids. How are these poor teachers supposed to keep their students focused throughout the day? SO frustrated! And, that is my rant for the day!!!

Each of these government-sponsored food-like-substances contain between nine and 16 grams of sugar per serving (without factoring in any syrup for the French toast or pancakes), with all but one coming from high fructose corn syrup. One gram of sugar contains 3.87 calories, which means this government-sponsored "breakfast" served up between 34.83 and 61.92 calories of pure sugar (or roughly 50% of what the American Heart Association believes to be a "safe" daily allotment) to kids just before their brains were going to be called to action.

Each of these food-like-substances *also contains* GMOs (and therefore most likely pesticides) and gluten and were most likely accompanied by a serving of milk, each of which will be discussed further in following chapters.

---

[x] http://articles.mercola.com/sites/articles/archive/2014/02/04/modern-diet.aspx; March 11, 2014.

[xi] http://www.usda.gov/factbook/chapter2.pdf; March 11, 2014.

[xii] http://archinte.jamanetwork.com/article.aspx?articleid=1819573; March 11, 2014.

[xiii] Effects of soft drink consumption on nutrition and health: a systematic review and meta-analysis. http://geti.in/17ErkaX; March 11, 2014.

[xiv] http://articles.mercola.com/sites/articles/archive/2013/07/24/diet-soda-dangers.aspx; March 11, 2014.

[xv] http://articles.mercola.com/sites/articles/archive/2013/07/24/diet-soda-dangers.aspx; March 11, 2014.

[xvi] http://archive.sciencewatch.com/inter/aut/2010/10-nov/10novCant/; March 11, 2014.

[xvii] http://www.foodaddictionsummit.org/docs/SticeSpoor2008.pdf; March 11, 2014.

CHAPTER 2

GENETICALLY MODIFIED ORGANISMS (GMOs)

Genetically Modified Organisms (GMOs) are created when genes from one species (e.g. from a fly or a toxin such as BT-toxin) are forced into the DNA of another species (e.g. tomatoes or corn). While it may sound like a Frankenstein science experiment, both of these examples are real. The Food and Drug Administration (FDA) has approved and allowed genes from flies to be crossed with tomatoes and BT-toxin to be crossed with corn. These foods, the GMO tomatoes and corn, as well as others, are allowed to be fed to our children daily on school campuses across North America. But it doesn't stop there.

Most Common Genetically Modified Foods

Eighty percent of corn and soy crops in North America have been engineered to withstand normally deadly doses of herbicides, primarily Monsanto's Roundup. GMO corn varieties are also engineered to produce their own toxic insecticide that breaks open the stomach of insects and kills them.

There are some genetically modified foods that are so pervasive, so common, that they are found as fillers in just about any product you pick up off of the packaged and/or "prepared foods" shelves. You would need to be super diligent and read labels, including those on fresh fruits, vegetables, meat, dairy and poultry that you buy.

Oh, did I forget to mention? The agricultural industry has thus far been successful in preventing a law that would require GMO labeling. That's right, companies currently don't have to tell you whether their products were made using (or animals fed with) genetically modified organisms. Thankfully, however, there are movements happening that are encouraging the voluntary labeling and certification of foods that are "non-GMO."

The 5 most common GMOs

- soybeans
- canola
- cottonseed
- corn
- sugar from sugar beet

If you consume animal products (beef, chicken, pork, eggs, milk, etc.), you could still be exposed to the GMOs because of the feed used for these animals. Most factory farming operations in North America are now using GMO-feed or GMO-tainted-feed on their livestock. It is possible to buy organic, grass-fed meat, dairy and eggs, but you have to ask your grocers or farmers specifically about the products that you are buying. You can be certain that school cafeterias do not certify that the foods served to your children are non-GMO or organic (at least not yet!).

What's the big deal? If Genetically Modified Organisms are in just about everything, does it really matter? Yes. Genetically modified plants either drink poison or produce poison. Then, we eat those plants OR the animals (or their products) that ate those plants. Roundup, an insecticide now found in the blood of pregnant women and their unborn children, has been found to be extremely dangerous.[xviii] Multiple independent studies raise questions about links to allergies and other serious potential health risks including cancer.[xix]

Genetically modified foods have been suspected to be involved in various health related issues: Gastro-intestinal disorders, allergies, asthma, auto-immune conditions, skin rashes and acne, brain fog, reproductive disorders, acid reflux, energy, weight gain, and more. These same disorders (e.g. reproductive, immune and GI tract) have been reported among livestock and lab animals fed GMOs. There also remains a significant question: when we consume a genetically modified organism, does it alter our own or our children's DNA? This and other critical questions were *never asked or answered* before the USDA and FDA allowed these foods to be produced and served to our children at school.

Why don't we hear more about this and why have we been told just the opposite, that GMOs are safe?

Because GMOs represent a multi-billion dollar investment by chemical and agricultural companies. They would like to make all plants GMO so that they can legally patent and "own" the seeds. It has thus far not been possible for independent research to be done on GMO seeds and the companies holding the patents on them have refused to allow open and unbiased (independent) research (and have controlled the release of all data and reporting on genetically modified organisms).

There have never been human studies with *any* of the GMO foods.

Despite this, the American Academy of Environmental Medicine (AAEM) urges all doctors to prescribe non-GMO diets for their patients. What we do have are rising rates of digestive and immune conditions (all of which can be tied back to the gut, a disabling of beneficial gut bacteria and micronutrients). "Elimination diets," diets where specific foods are pulled out to see how a patient responds, don't lie. If a food is removed and all symptoms go away, it is highly likely that the food was the culprit. Many physicians now prescribe non-GMO diets, and people are getting better from a variety of disorders. Livestock taken off GMOs are also getting better.

Our children are not guinea pigs. If there is *any chance* that GMO foods are causing digestive and immune conditions or any other harm, they should not be allowed in or on our school campuses!

xviii http://www.scientificamerican.com/article/weed-whacking-herbicide-p/; March 15, 2014.

xix http://responsibletechnology.org/docs/gmos-are-not-safe.pdf; March 15, 2014.

CHAPTER 3

PESTICIDES, HERBICIDES AND INSECTICIDES

While processed fructose (high fructose corn syrup, specifically) wins top billing as the "greatest destroyer of health," I am suspicious that the reason for that includes the fact that almost *all* of the corn used to make the high fructose corn syrup has been either sprayed or genetically modified with pesticides, herbicides and/or insecticides.

Pesticides, herbicides and insecticides are discussed following the GMO chapter because they stem from the same source (chemical companies) and they are becoming increasingly difficult to separate. Pesticide, insecticide, fungicide, herbicide—"cidal" substances—are made to kill and they are indiscriminate. An herbicide will kill plants. Insecticides and fungicides are mitochondrial disruptors— that is, they cause dysfunction and cell death of mitochondria (more on that later).

It used to be that pesticides, herbicides and insecticides were sprayed *on* a plant or a weed to either detract insects or kill an unwanted plant/weed. Since the process of genetic modification has come about, there have been some companies that are not just spraying; they are putting the chemicals *in* the plants (e.g., BT-corn).

For the longest time we were told that there was no increased risk to consumers exposed to or regularly eating crops sprayed with pesticides and/or insecticides. History has shown that to have been a lie and most agencies overseeing pesticides agree that they pose a risk, especially to infants and children.[xx]

Infants and children are more sensitive to the toxic effects of pesticides than adults.

- An infant's brain, nervous system, and organs are still developing after birth.

- When exposed, a baby's immature liver and kidneys cannot remove pesticides from the body as well as an adult's liver and kidneys.

- Infants may also be exposed to more pesticide than adults because they take more breaths per minute and have more skin surface relative to their body weight.

- Children often spend more time closer to the ground, touching baseboards and lawns where pesticides may have been applied.

- Children often eat and drink more relative to their body weight than adults, which can lead to a higher dose of pesticide residue per pound of body weight.

- Babies that crawl on treated carpeting may have a greater potential to dislodge pesticide residue onto their skin or breathe in pesticide-laden dust.

- Young children are also more likely to put their fingers, toys, and other objects into their mouths.

The Environmental Protection Agency (EPA) states that, "Pesticides may harm a developing child by blocking the absorption of important food nutrients necessary for normal healthy growth. Another way pesticides may cause harm is if a child's excretory system is not fully developed, the body may not fully remove pesticides. Also, there are 'critical periods' in human development when exposure to a toxin can permanently alter the way an individual's biological system operates."[xxi] The American Academy of Pediatrics (AAP) has reported that "epidemiologic evidence demonstrates associations between early life exposure to pesticides and pediatric cancers, decreased cognitive function, and behavioral problems."[xxii]

Chemicals are liberally applied in and around the school environment as well as being found in the food supply. During 2014-15 school registration, parents in one district were handed an 8 ½" x 11" piece of paper with a solid list (about a 10 pt. font) of all of the chemicals that are applied inside and outside of the school buildings. Just as a warning, so we can say we told you. But what are we supposed to do about it? And where is that same list to warn us about all of the chemicals that they are allowing in the food?

Roundup is an herbicide and was patented as a potent biocidal: an antimicrobial that knocks out organisms. Research data in cattle and chickens is showing that Roundup (active ingredient glyphosate) is knocking out some of the beneficial gut bacteria. Our stomach and intestinal tracts (aka "gut") make up 60-85% of our total immune system. If the gut isn't healthy, the body isn't healthy. It is responsible for the majority of inflammation, diseases and autoimmune conditions.

Allergies are the *first* sign that the gut flora is not healthy.

BT-toxin is designed to create a crystal-based protein that disrupts the mitochondria of insects. Mitochondria are what line our intestinal tract. This toxin has been genetically engineered to grow *inside of* corn. So when an insect eats the corn, the toxin causes the disruption of mitochondria, which kills them. This toxin is bio-accumulating in humans and no research has ever been done to show what would happen to our intestinal lining as a result. There are some hypotheses that some of the cause of increased leaky gut (causing increases in food allergies and overall inflammation) in our population may be because of the bioaccumulation of these toxins.

Despite the knowledge that pesticides, herbicides and insecticides pose a risk, there have been NO regulations for pesticides and other chemicals in and on school campuses.

There have also been no regulations on the chemical Roundup (as in, to make sure that it's not so extensively used that it ends up in our water and food supply). A study in Quebec showed that 93% of pregnant women and 80% of their unborn offspring had elevated levels of (the crystal-based proteins) BT-toxin circulating in their blood. And 100% of their unborn fetuses had glyphosate (the herbicide).

In children, it was found that "diet may be the most influential source [of pesticide exposure]." An intervention study placed children on an organic diet (produced without pesticide) and observed a drastic and immediate decrease in urinary excretion of pesticide metabolites.[xxiii] Organic diets significantly lower children's dietary exposure to organophosphorus pesticides.[xxiv]

Pesticide Residues in Produce

The produce ranking (shown in the following tables) developed by analysts at Environmental Working Group (EWG), is based on the results of nearly 51,000 tests for pesticide residues on produce collected by the U.S. Department of Agriculture and the U.S. Food and Drug Administration.

Dirty Dozen™ 2014

Apples	Peaches
Celery	Potatoes
Cherry Tomatoes	Snap peas (imported)
Cucumbers	Spinach
Grapes	Strawberries
Nectarines (imported)	Sweet bell peppers

Plus

Hot Peppers	Kale/Collards

The list has been updated for 2014. EWG is a not-for-profit environmental research organization dedicated to improving public health and protecting the environment. You can learn more about them and their work at www.ewg.org.

The Clean Fifteen™ 2014

Asparagus	Mangoes
Avocados	Onions
Cabbage	Papayas
Cantaloupe	Pineapples
Cauliflower	Sweet corn
Eggplant	Sweet peas (frozen)
Grapefruit	Sweet potatoes
Kiwi	

A good recommendation is to use these lists to shop for your produce, in order to diminish your risks from pesticide-related health problems. For instance, if a fruit or vegetable resides on the Dirty

Dozen™ list, you should try to buy it organically. But if budgets are tight and you find a fruit or vegetable from The Clean Fifteen™ list that is not organic, you are more likely to be safe with the amount of chemicals typically found on these types of produce.

Apples are the most common fruit offered to kids through the school lunch program and yet they are consistently *the most contaminated* fruit and/or vegetable. Shouldn't that dictate that *only organic* apples should be purchased for students' consumption on school campuses? Why do we allow schools to offer our children *the most contaminated* foods? This is unacceptable!

It is clear that the alphabet soup of government agencies (EPA, FDA and USDA), who were supposed to protect us, are *not talking to each other* about how foods hurt us (EPA), the chemicals that they are allowing *on and in* our food (FDA) and *what* they are allowing to be served on school campuses (USDA). In addition, the present medical field was not trained or equipped with how to test and treat chemical and pesticide toxicity. Nor is there sufficient regulatory action on pesticide use (including the use *in* the food). There is no current reliable way to determine the incidence of pesticide exposure and illness in US children. All we have are the growing list of "unexplainable" illnesses that are skyrocketing over the last few decades: autism, ADHD, asthma, allergies, childhood obesity, early onset of Type 2 diabetes, childhood symptoms of hypertension, metabolic syndrome, early cancers and more.

We are now finding symptoms in children (and adults) that cannot be distinguished between pesticides, herbicides, insecticides or GMO-foods. Some were discussed in the previous chapter. The solution is the same. When the food is removed and the symptom

24

clears up, it is logical that the food was the problem. The recommendation: remove all pesticides, insecticides and GMO-foods from your (and your children's) diet.

[xx] http://npic.orst.edu/health/child.html; available March 21, 2014
[xxi] http://www.epa.gov/pesticides/food/pest.htm; available August 25, 2014
[xxii] http://pediatrics.aappublications.org/content/130/6/e1757.full; available March 21, 2014
[xxiii] Lu C, Toepel K, Irish R, Fenske RA, Barr DB, Bravo R. Organic diets significantly lower children's dietary exposure to organophosphorus pesticides. Environ Health Perspect. 2006;114(2):260–263.
[xxiv] Environ Health Perspect. 2006;114(2):260–263]

CHAPTER 4

GLUTEN

Wheat, more than any other food-like item (including sugar), is woven into the fabric of the American diet. It has become seemingly essential: toast for breakfast, sandwiches for lunch, bagels, hamburger and hot dog buns, and pasta. Wheat, by a considerable margin is the dominant source of gluten in the North American diet.

Gluten is a protein found not only in wheat, but also in related grain species, including barley and rye (and food processed from these grains). Gluten gives elasticity to dough, helping it rise and keep its shape and often gives the final product a chewy texture. Gluten is also used in many cosmetics, hair products and other dermatological preparations.[xxv]

There has been a debate whether many reported increases in gluten-sensitive conditions (Celiac Disease, Non-Celiac-Gluten-Sensitivity and Irritable Bowel Syndrome) are due to the changes in the wheat itself or due to the pesticides and chemicals that have been used on our wheat for the past few decades. Either way, it has been causing great harm in a large number of people.

Modern wheat is not the same kind of wheat that your grandparents ate.

The nutritional content of this staple grain has been dramatically altered over the past 50+ years and is now far less nutritious than previous varieties. As Kris Gunnars reports, "Modern dwarf wheat was introduced around the year 1960, which contains 19-28 percent less of important minerals like Magnesium, Iron, Zinc, and Copper.

There is also evidence that modern wheat is much more harmful to celiac patients and people with gluten sensitivity, compared to older breeds like Einkorn wheat. Whereas whole, unprocessed, wheat may have been relatively healthy back in the day, the same is not true of modern dwarf wheat."[xxvi,xxvii] Today's wheat has a much higher concentration of gluten, making the digestibility more much difficult.

Dr. Mercola reports that wheat lectin (or *wheat germ agglutinin*) is largely responsible for many of the problems that wheat creates in our bodies. He further states, "[Lectin] is highest in whole wheat, especially sprouted whole wheat, but wheat isn't the only grain with significant lectin. All seeds of the grass family (rice, wheat, spelt, rye, etc.) are high in lectins.

Lectin has the potential to damage your health by the following mechanisms (list is not all-inclusive):"[xxviii]

- **Pro-Inflammatory:** Lectin stimulates the synthesis of pro-inflammatory chemical messengers, even at very small concentrations.

- **Neurotoxic:** Lectin can pass through your blood-brain barrier and attach to the protective coating on your nerves, known as the myelin sheath. It is also capable of inhibiting nerve growth factor, which is important for the growth, maintenance, and survival of certain neurons.

- **Immunotoxic:** Lectin may bind to and activate white blood cells.

- **Cardiotoxic:** Lectin induces platelet aggregation and has a potent disruptive effect on tissue regeneration and the removal of neutrophils from your blood vessels.

- **Cytotoxic (toxic to cells):** Lectin may induce programmed cell death (apoptosis).

- Research also shows that lectin may **disrupt endocrine and gastrointestinal function, interfere with genetic expression**, and share similarities with certain viruses

There is *no risk* to avoiding gluten, but the potential risks of consuming it keeps growing. Dr. Alessio Fasano (head of the Department of Pediatric Gastroenterology and Nutrition at Massachusetts General Hospital for Children) says that "gluten is not digestible by any human kind." He clarifies that this poor digestibility may not have a consequence in some, but it has clearly posed a dire consequence for others. He goes on to say that "gluten is, nutritionally speaking, useless." It has no purpose to our well-being.

Conditions helped by removing gluten from the diet include:

- ADD/ADHD
- Anxiety and chronic stress
- Chronic headaches and migraines
- Depression
- Diabetes
- Epilepsy
- Focus and concentration problems
- Inflammatory conditions and disease, including arthritis
- Insomnia
- Intestinal problems, including celiac disease, gluten sensitivity and irritable bowel syndrome
- Memory problems and mild cognitive impairment
- Mood disorders

- Overweight and obesity
- Tourette's syndrome[xxix]

If this list weren't bad enough, research has also shown that gluten disrupts our body's pH balance (the thing used by our immune system to fight disease, including cancer) and accelerates the process of aging through advanced glycation end products (causes arteries to harden, cataracts to form, dementia and wrinkling of the skin). Phew!

So why, you ask, is gluten so pervasive and again, why haven't we heard more about it? I'll give you a hint: Industry and profit. We have been "advertised" to by the USDA, the Whole Grain Council, the Whole Wheat Council, the American Dietetic Association, the American Diabetes Association, and the American Heart Association, to "eat more healthy whole grains" and wheat is what we were offered. Their industries are built upon our eating more.

We were and are told, and our children are instructed in school, to eat *more* of this potentially dangerous protein. But cutting it out, after a lifetime of programming and food habits, can be very hard. I get it! You might be saying, "What, no wheat? What will I eat? I'll starve!" Let me say it again, I get it! My family has been there and it's a journey. In the last section of the book, What Can Parents Do, I try to outline a plan of action and provide resources to help you navigate these new waters. It may be difficult to make change, but your body (and your brain) will thank you!!

[xxv] Harding, Anne (October 31, 2011). http://thechart.blogs.cnn.com/2011/10/31/gluten-in-cosmetics-may-pose-hidden-threat-to-celiac-patients/. Retrieved March 11, 2014.
[xxvi] http://www.ncbi.nlm.nih.gov/pmc/articles/PMC2963738/, available March 20, 2014.
[xxvii]
http://informahealthcare.com/doi/abs/10.1080/00365520600699983?journalCo

de=gas&, Retrieved March 20, 2014.

xxviii http://articles.mercola.com/sites/articles/archive/2014/02/24/modern-diet.aspx, Retrieved March 20, 2014.

xxix Perlmutter MD, David, Grain Brain: The Surprising Truth about Wheat, Carbs, and Sugar—Your Brain's Silent Killers, Little, Brown and Company, 2013.

CHAPTER 5

DAIRY

The topic of dairy, and the chance that it might be harmful, brings up deep emotional feelings in many of us. After all, we were raised to believe (and repeatedly told by attractive celebrities donning milk mustaches) that their product would "do our body good." As with wheat, the modern dairy products available in supermarkets today are nothing like they used to be. Today's milk looks the same, but it is not the same nutritionally.

The Increase in Dairy Consumption

Cheese in history: surprisingly when many Americans think of dairy, they only think of milk. They shudder to put cheese in the same harmful category. Cheese, has caseomorphins which literally make it addicting! In the U.S., cheese consumption increased 180 percent between 1970 and 2003 and cheese is the primary source of saturated fat in our diet. We went from eating 3.8 pounds of cheese per person in 1900 to 31.4 pounds per person in 2005.[xxx] With the creation and rise of fast food restaurants, cheeseburgers and pizza became commonplace, spurring the massive increase in cheese consumption.

No studies have shown that consuming dairy prevents disease. Conversely, numerous studies have shown that it contributes to diseases, including prostate cancer,[xxxi,xxxii,xxxiii,xxxiv,xxxv] increased rates of hip fracture,[xxxvi,xxxvii] as well as difficulties in metabolism for people with specific gene mutations, contributing to methylation and sulfation pathway disruption (both methylation and sulfation disruptions are commonly found in children with autism and auto-immune conditions).

The bottom line: there is an industry, represented by the Dairy Council, which makes money off of these products. They have and will continue to fight for survival and "market share." In America, the dairy industry is heavily subsidized through Farm Bill appropriations (congressional subsidies, using tax payer money). We pay for it to be produced and over-consumed by Americans.

The Dairy Council is one of the largest, and most subsidized, industries that exists around our food. They have lobbied very heavily to keep a "separate" food category for themselves on the USDA's *Dietary Guidelines for America* (currently known as *MyPlate*) despite the fact that dairy is, after all, just another animal food source of protein (and some carbohydrate). Current *MyPlate* recommendations include three glasses of milk per day *for everyone* (no disclosure of potential long term risks for a large portion of the population).

The Dairy Council will fight aggressively against any statements made in this or any other book or article that speaks about any negative health effects from dairy products (just dismissing, maligning or paying to "crowd it out"). But remember (Buyer Beware!) only you are looking out for your personal and family's health. When in doubt, try an elimination diet. If removing dairy (*all dairy*) helps alleviate your high cholesterol, headaches, allergies, acne or other problems, then it was an irritant in *your* body and needs to be removed, permanently.

There is a movement promoting the return of non-homogenized milk. It is still available directly from dairies in some states, but in others it is illegal. There is insufficient research, in my opinion, to substantiate *health benefits* of non-homogenized milk nor is there research to show it does not initiate some of the health risks shown with homogenized milk (hip fractures, cancer promotion, metabolic disruption, etc.). I leave this call up to you and your decisions for the health of your family.

I follow the tenet and oath, even with food, that medical doctors were once asked to take and follow: "first do no harm." If there is research that shows a food can cause harm *and* there is no research showing that it actually produces healthy outcomes, I'm not going to risk it with my family *nor should our schools with our children*! In our family, we have removed dairy completely and replaced milk with coconut, almond and/or hemp milk, which can be purchased in stores or made at home. There are even some *super* tasty nut cheeses that we use sparingly when entertaining people who aren't used to our way of eating (they often cannot even tell the difference!).

HISTORICAL SUMMARY[xxxviii]

1600s and 1700s: a cow yielded approximately one quart of milk per day. Cream was churned into butter and was stored to help provide nourishment during the winter.

1908: Pasteurization was introduced to reduce spoiling and the growth of bacteria.

1919: Homogenization began to prevent the separation of fat.

1932: Synthetic Vitamin D was first added to milk.

1964: Plastic milk containers are first commercially introduced.

1994: Monsanto develops the genetically engineered growth hormone, recombinant bovine somatotropin (rBST) or bovine growth hormone (BGH) to boost dairy yield.

Pasteurization - boiling the milk kills any bacteria, but it also affects the taste and nutritional value. Translation: it also kills the vitamins. As a result, they now add a few back in (fortified) after the fact. However, many of those vitamins and minerals added back in afterwards are synthetic and not even usable by our bodies (this fortification principle applies to many other foods that have been denatured from their original form and "human-improved" as well).

Homogenization - milk is pushed through a fine filter at pressures of ~4,000 pounds per square inch; the fat globules are made smaller by a factor of ten times or more; these fat molecules then become evenly dispersed throughout the milk so they stay integrated rather than separating as cream.

Milk is a hormonal delivery system. When homogenized, milk becomes very powerful and efficient at bypassing normal digestive processes and delivering steroid and protein hormones to the human body (both your hormones and the cow's natural hormones and the ones they may have been injected with to produce more milk).

Homogenization makes fat molecules in milk smaller and they become "capsules" for substances that are able to bypass digestion. Proteins that would normally be digested in the stomach are not broken down and instead they are absorbed into the bloodstream. Studies have shown that these protein-heavy fat globules can potentially increase homogenized milk's ability to cause allergic reactions (or sensitivities; an IgG response which causes inflammation in the gut). Other known effects on milk quality include increased viscosity (the milk is thickened in consistency), whiter appearance, lowered heat stability, increased sensitivity to light-triggered oxidation and less pronounced milk flavor.

The homogenization process breaks up an enzyme in milk which in its smaller state can then enter the bloodstream and react against arterial walls. This causes the body to protect the area with a layer of cholesterol. If this only happened once in a while it would not be a big concern, but if it happens regularly there are long term risks: inflammation leading to higher levels of cholesterol and atherosclerosis (or clogging of the arteries).

Proteins were created to be easily broken down by digestive processes. Homogenization disrupts this and ensures their survival so that they enter the bloodstream. Many times the body reacts to foreign proteins by producing histamines, and then mucus. Sometimes homogenized milk proteins resemble a human protein and can become triggers for autoimmune diseases such as diabetes or multiple sclerosis.

Two Connecticut cardiologists (Oster & Ross) have demonstrated that homogenized milk proteins did in fact survive digestion. It was discovered that Bovine Xanthene Oxidase (BXO) survived long enough to affect every one of three hundred heart attack victims over a five-year time period. Even young children in the U.S. are showing signs of hardening of the arteries.^{xxxix}

Lactose (sugar) intolerance – this can occur when someone does not have the enzyme lipase needed to break down the lactose sugar molecule; these individuals can supplement the enzyme lipase and still tolerate many dairy products.

Casein or whey sensitivity or allergy – as opposed to lactose, which is the carbohydrate (sugar molecule) in dairy, casein and whey are the proteins. You can be allergic (or sensitive) to either one or both of the proteins.

- A Type 1 food allergy can occur when your body's immune system mistakenly thinks the protein is harmful and inappropriately produces **IgE antibodies** for protection (occurs in less than 5% of the population; usually children). Symptoms can be immediate and include stomach cramping, diarrhea, skin rashes, hives, swelling, wheezing or the most dreaded of Type 1 reactions, anaphylaxis.

- **Type 3 immune reactions are much more common, but are often dismissed by medical doctors and therefore schools!** They occur when your immune system creates an overabundance of **IgG antibodies** to a particular food. The IgG antibodies, instead of attaching to mast cells like IgE antibodies in Type 1 allergies, bind directly to the food as it enters the bloodstream, forming different sizes of so-called circulating immune complexes (food allergens bound to antibodies circulating in the bloodstream). In an IgG reaction, the IgG antibodies attach themselves to the food antigen and create an antibody-antigen complex. These complexes are normally removed by special cells called macrophages. However, if they are present in large numbers and the reactive food is still being consumed, the macrophages cannot remove them quickly enough. The food antigen-antibody complexes accumulate and are deposited in body tissues. Once in the tissue, these complexes release inflammation causing chemicals, which may play a role in numerous diseases and conditions. **Translation: continued**

35

consumption of a food with an IgG reaction causes inflammation in the gut and other body tissues, leading to disease!

Antibiotics - 80% of antibiotics used globally are in animals that become our food. Increased use of growth hormones (rBST or BGH) causes increased utter infections, an increased need for antibiotics, as well as resultant pus in the milk. It was also discussed in the chapter about pesticides, herbicides and insecticides how Roundup (active ingredient glyphosate) is knocking out beneficial gut bacteria in cattle (as well as in chickens). This would put the animals at greater risk of lowered immunity, causing an increased need again, for antibiotics (or ideally a longer term solution like healing their guts, their natural immunity and the quality of their meat).

Hormones - are given to dairy cows to promote growth, reproduction (make them have repeated pregnancies) and to increase milk production. Synthetic hormones, rBST or BGH, are now used in the U.S. but are banned in Canada, parts of the E.U., Australia and New Zealand.

Pesticides/Herbicides/Insecticides - in larger dairies, lactating animals can be treated with insecticides by daily or every-other-day coat sprays. In addition, the food supply given to most dairy cows is heavily sprayed with Roundup or other chemicals, which are now being found in the blood and fetuses of pregnant women.

Gene mutations and metabolism – people that have a common gene mutation that inhibits methylation pathways have an increased susceptibility to IgG reactions to gluten and dairy, which lead to increased inflammation in the gut and a decreased uptake of consumed nutrients. Those with this mutation who consume dairy have an increased risk of folate receptor blocking autoantibody production.[xl] Long term this can also contribute to a toxic build-up as the pathways get blocked.

Role of dairy in school food programs

In 1946 the National School Lunch Act was passed. The legislation was identified as the "National School Lunch Act," and Section 2 of the Act defines its purposes: "It is hereby declared to be the policy of Congress, as a measure of national security, to safeguard the health and well-being of the Nation's children and to encourage the domestic consumption of nutritious agricultural commodities and other food, by assisting the States, through grants-in aid and other means, in providing an adequate supply of food and other facilities for the establishment, maintenance, operation and expansion of nonprofit school lunch programs."[xli]

The next part is what bothers me the most: Section 9 of the Act provided that "Lunches served by schools participating in the school lunch program under this Act shall meet minimum nutritional requirements prescribed by the Secretary **on the basis of tested nutritional research**." And you can bet that no independent research followed. Despite much research that has shown that dairy has questionable and even harmful effects in many people, especially long term, and many amendments to the National School Lunch Act and the inclusion now of the School Breakfast program, dairy remains an integral part of these programs to this very day.

When I advised the public school that my children were attending in 1998 that they had milk allergies, I was told that no other beverage options were available to children at lunch unless a doctor's note was provided. I promptly provided such a note but was a bit miffed that not even water was offered as a viable option *by choice.* My children continued to be offered milk every single day at lunch and had to repeatedly say **"no"** and ask for their other option (allowable under the allergy exemption). To this day young people have to be vocal about desiring options other than milk. Some schools now have a pitcher of tap water available for kids from which to pour a glass. I feel like nutritionally we're still living in the Stone Age (research be darned)!

[xxx] USDA Economic Research Service. Dietary Assessment of Major Trends in U.S. Food Consumption.1970-2005.

http://www.ers.usda.gov/media/210681/eib33_1_.pdf

[xxxi] Howell MA. Factor analysis of international cancer mortality data and per capita food consumption. Br J Cancer. 1974;29:328-336.

[xxxii] Armstrong B, Doll R. Environmental factors and cancer incidence and mortality in different countries, with special reference to dietary practices. Int J Cancer. 1975;15: 617-631.

[xxxiii] Rose DP, Boyar AP, Wynder EL. International comparisons of mortality rates for cancer of the breast, ovary, prostate, and colon, and per capita food consumption. Cancer. 1986;58:2363-2371.

[xxxiv] Decarli A, La Vecchia C. Environmental factors and cancer mortality in Italy: correlational exercise. Oncology. 1986;43:116-126.

[xxxv] Hebert JR, Hurley TG, Olendzki BC, Teas J, Ma Y, Hampl JS. Nutritional and socioeconomic factors in relation to prostate cancer mortality: a cross national study. J Natl Cancer Inst. 1998;90(21):1637-1647.

[xxxvi] Cumming, RG. "Case-control study of risk factors for hip fractures in the elderly." Am J Epidemiol. 1994 Mar 1;139(5):493-503.

[xxxvii] Warensjo E, Byberg L, Melhus H, et al. Dietary calcium intake and risk of fracture and osteoporosis: prospective longitudinal cohort study. BMJ. 2011;342:d1473.

[xxxviii] www.naturalnews.com/022967_milk_pasteurization_dairy.html#; available April 2, 2014

[xxxix] http://www.naturalnews.com/022967_milk_pasteurization_dairy.html#; available April 2, 2014

[xl] Berrocal-Zaragoza MI, Murphy MM, Ceruelo S, Quadros EV, Sequeira JM, Fernandez-Ballart JD. High milk consumers have an increased risk of folate receptor blocking autoantibody production but this does not affect folate status in Spanish men and women. J Nutr 2009b;139:1037-1041.

[xli] P L. 396 -79th Congress, June 4, 1946, 60 Stat. 231.

CHAPTER 6

FAT vs. OIL AND IMBALANCES OF ESSENTIAL FATTY ACIDS

Dietary fat (the stuff we eat), together with carbohydrates and protein (collectively called the *macro*nutrients), plays an essential role in our diet and health. It provides energy, absorbs certain nutrients, lubricates joints and nerves and maintains the core body temperature. Fats are especially important for children for proper growth and development (including the brain). While fat (from natural whole foods) is essential, oil (a processed version of a plant) is not. And the kind of fat you eat is *really* what matters.

The government and other organizations have primarily focused on the caloric density of fat (with fat providing more calories than either carbohydrate or protein ounce-for-ounce). In addition, they have erroneously blamed fat alone for high cholesterol levels. Nearly all U.S. healthcare organizations (e.g. American Dietetic Association, American Diabetes Association, American Heart Association and National Cancer Institute) have largely ignored the *function and quality* of dietary fats and simply recommended an overall "decreased intake."

As a result, back in the '80s, there was a fad to go "low fat" in everything. All they did was water a product down to decrease the "percent of fat" but because it lost some flavor in the process, often sugar was added in place of the fat. And they did some creative math on the labels. But research would show that Americans never really did "lower" their fat intake, as fat intake per person in the U.S. has gone up consistently since 1970 (some suggest our increased intake of cheese surpassed our attempts to decrease fat in other foods). But intake from added sugar and white flour went up even faster (that, however, is discussed in another chapter)!

So what is it about fat that makes it healthy or unhealthy in our diets and bodies? It's the type and amount of fatty acid found in food that determines the effect of the fat on your health.

From a functional perspective, not all fat (even fat within the same classifications), is the same. Typically fats are classified as either saturated, unsaturated or trans fatty acids.

Classification of Fats:

- **Saturated fats** (or fatty acids) can come from plant or animal sources and can be short, medium or long chain fatty acids.

- **Unsaturated fatty acids** are classified as Omega 3, Omega 6 or Omega 9. While Omega 9 fatty acids can be synthesized in our body from saturated fat, Omega 3 and 6 cannot, so they are called essential fatty acids, meaning we have an "essential" need to obtain Omega 3 and Omega 6 fatty acids from our food.**Trans fatty acids** are created. That's right. They are not found in nature and are only found in man-made oils and food products. The food industry has increased the solidification of plant oils by adding a nickel catalyst to them, heating them, passing hydrogen through them, rebleaching them, and then removing the nickel catalyst by filtration. This process is called hydrogenation and has zero health benefit and has proven to be harmful.

What these simple classifications fail to tell you is how each of those is further broken down as to function in the body. Macronutrients, including fat, have typically been simply looked at for their singular function of energy production. What other roles does fat have in our body?

- Different fatty acid "shapes" (and composition) regulate different cell membranes; in the brain, 35 percent of cell membrane "fats" contain an Omega 3 fatty acid; in the eye, photoreceptor "fats" may contain up to 60 percent of an Omega 3 fatty acid; in infants and children, changes in fatty acid composition, especially Omega 3 fatty acid deficiencies, have been suggested to contribute to conditions such as attention deficit and hyperactivity disorder (ADD and ADHD)[xlii] and may influence visual capacity.[xliii]

- It has been shown that **insufficient levels of essential fatty acids (Omega 3 and 6) are one of the most significant nutritional factors in the etiology of cardiovascular disease.**[xliv]

- There is a desired ratio of Omega 6 to Omega 3 fatty acids for optimum health. Most researchers agree that it is about a 2:1 ratio. The maintenance of this ratio appears to play a critical role in a wide variety of health conditions, including:

    o Cancer

    o Skin-related disorders

    o Immune-related disorders

    o Endocrine-related disorders

    o Cardiovascular disorders

    o General inflammatory conditions

- Omega 6 fatty acids compete for enzymes that convert both Omega 6 and Omega 3 into anti-inflammatory substances. **Therefore, an excess intake of Omega 6 fatty acids, even in the presence of Omega 3 fatty acids, may render the Omega 3s silent.**

So, even the essential fatty acids Omega 3 and Omega 6 are "needed" in *different quantities*. As mentioned previously, nutrients in food cannot be studied in isolation. There is rarely a food that contains only one type of nutrient and it is the dynamic interaction of these nutrients that benefit our health. Well, it's the same with the essential fatty acids. Whole plant foods tend to contain a balance of Omega 3 and 6 fats ... and uniquely, that balance tends to be in a ratio that our body needs. But here are foods that are "higher" in either one or the other of the essential fatty acids:

- Omega 3s are highest in cold-water fish (salmon, halibut and sardines) and are also found in flax seeds, black currant and walnuts and to a lesser extent even in Brussel sprouts, kale, spinach, and salad greens and oils (flaxseed, walnut, salmon, cod liver and canola).*

- Omega 6s are highest in grain-fed animal products (meat, milk, eggs), poppy seeds, wheat germ, sesame, sunflower and pumpkin seeds, pine nuts, pecans, avocados and oils (safflower, grape seed, corn, peanut and olive).*

When receiving fatty acids from oils, you get a concentrated dose, but you miss all of the other balanced nutrients that were found in the natural whole plant with those essential oils. When possible, eat the whole plant rather than using it in an oil form.

The problem comes when we receive a majority of our daily fat intake from oil and animal sources rather than whole, plant-based foods. Because in doing so, we are likely to have an imbalance of the essential fatty acids.

The increased consumption of processed vegetable oils and grain-fed meats has led to a severely lopsided fatty acid composition, as these provide high amounts of Omega 6 fats. The ideal ratio of Omega 6 to Omega 3 fats is 2:1 (or even a modest 4:1), but the typical Western diet, *including food served on school campuses*, is between 30:1 and 50:1! Eating these fats out of balance sets the stage for cardiovascular disease, cancer, depression and Alzheimer's, rheumatoid arthritis and diabetes.[xlv]

To correct this Omega 6 to Omega 3 fatty acid imbalance, two things need to occur:

1. Intake of Omega 6 foods needs to decrease greatly (processed foods, foods cooked at high temperatures using vegetable oils, grain-fed meat, eggs from grain-fed chickens, dairy from grain fed cattle)

2. Intake of Omega 3 foods needs to replace the Omega 6 foods (grass-fed organic meats and eggs, salmon and other cold-water fish, flax seeds) and supplementation may be necessary for some people (clean source of Omega 3 fatty acid or Krill oil).

This discussion about fats barely even scratches the surface of the functional role of various fats in our body and especially the role of essential fatty acids and our health. There is still so much research that needs to be done and lessons that we can learn. In the meantime, we know enough to disregard the simple message to "minimize fat intake." Rather, the message should be:

Eat to obtain the proper ratio of essential fatty acids, focus on whole foods, and avoid *all* trans fatty acids!

[xlii] Stevens LJ et all. Essential fatty acid metabolism in boys with attention-deficit hyperactivity disorder. Am J Clin Nutr. 1995 Oct;62(4):761-768.

[xliii] Hoffman DR et al. Effects of supplementation with omega 3 long-chain polyunsaturated fatty acids on retinal and cortical development in premature infants. Am J Clin Nutr. May 1993; 57(5 suppl):807S-812S.

[xliv] Siguel EN et al. Trans fatty acid metabolism in pateints with angiographically documented coronary artery disease. Am J Cardiol;71(11):916-920, 1993.

[xlv] http://articles.mercola.com/sites/articles/archive/2014/2/24/modern-diet.aspx

CHAPTER 7

ARTIFICIAL FOOD COLORINGS AND ADDITIVES

For years, food colorings and additives have been "added" to our food to either increase its marketing appeal (using pretty or at least more appealing colors), taste and/or shelf-life. However, this is another area where the Food and Drug Administration (FDA) has allowed something to be added to the food supply without providing independent research that says it is safe. And sadly, many food colorings and additives have caused harm. What the heck? Why isn't research being required *first* to ensure our safety?

So what are some of these "addings"? Well, you might remember the meat coloring scandal that was made public last year. As much as 70% of meat in grocery stores was being "gassed" to keep it red and make it appealing. Normally, once meat becomes exposed to air, oxidation begins which gradually turns the red color of the meat to a more unappetizing brown or grey color within just a few days. But the industrialized meat industry has been applying carbon monoxide, an odorless, colorless, poisonous gas (almost impossible to see, taste, or smell) in order to "make our meat look more appealing."

Or have you heard about beaver gland flavoring? Yes, you heard me right. *Castoreum* is a byproduct of the beaver's gland, added to their urine, which beavers use in nature to mark their territory. Well, food (and perfume) companies have found a way to add it to their products so that we eat (and wear) it. "Eeeeeeeew!" is right! These are just a couple that have hit public news in the past few years. What are some other things that are right under our noses or in our stomachs?

Food coloring – numbers and names have come and gone; for every one that they find to be carcinogenic, they just replace it with another one for a time. Why do they put food coloring in our food? Because we associate flavors with certain colors, food manufacturers use color to increase the perceived flavor enjoyment of food. Color additives are generally used for one of four specific reasons – to replace the color lost due to light exposure, storage, or temperature change; to add color to colorless foods; to correct natural color variations; or to enhance natural colors. Often manufacturers use a combination of several dyes to arrive at the color desired. Here are some of the current iterations of food coloring:

- **Blue Lake 1 or 2** - or anything that has "lake" in the name, are synthetic food coloring agents chemically synthesized from aromatic hydrocarbons derived from petroleum (yes, gas!); a chemical salt combined with a dye, allowing it to disperse in oil; **Blue Lake 1**, also called Brilliant Blue FCF, and **Blue Lake 2**, also called Indigo carmine; are used in baked goods, soaps, shampoos, cosmetics, toothpaste and mouthwash; *health risks are not clearly known*, but allergies have been linked and there are warnings against use during pregnancy. **Question: if it might cause harm to a developing fetus, wouldn't it also cause harm in a rapidly growing child?** Logical question to ask, but I guess no one cared to find out before they hoisted it on the public.

- **Red Lakes 2 and 3** are known to cause cancer, but were widely used for years before the FDA eventually banned them. We are now onto **Red Lakes 5-40** (no joke!) – used in maraschino cherries, canned fruits for salads, confections, baked goods, dairy products, snack foods, gelatin, contact lenses, beverages and more.

- **Green, Brown, Yellow, Orange and Violet Lakes** – used in beverages, puddings, ice cream, sherbet, cherries, confections, cereals, baked goods, snacks, dairy products, contact lenses, hotdog/sausage casings, toothpaste and more.

Caramel coloring – one of the oldest and single most-used food colorings in the world. Traditionally it was made from heated/oxidized sugar. Today it's mostly an artificial coloring that contains a potentially carcinogenic chemical called 4-methylimidazole (4-MeI). This coloring is commonly found in sodas, beer, many liquors, brown bread, buns, chocolate, cookies, cough drops, custards, decorations, fillings and toppings, potato chips, dessert mixes, doughnuts, fish and shellfish spreads, frozen desserts, fruit preserves, gravy, ice cream, pickles, sauces and dressings, vinegar, and more. Under California's new Proposition 65 law, any food or beverage sold in the state that exposes consumers to more than 29 micrograms of 4-MeI per day is supposed to carry a health-warning label (because it was found to be "possibly carcinogenic"). In recent *Consumer Reports*' tests, 12-ounce samples of Pepsi One and Malta Goya were found to have more than 29 micrograms per can or bottle and the California Attorney General has been asked to investigate. ***Buyer beware!***

Because this topic can be so "heavy," I thought I'd add some lightness by sharing some videos that might help you understand this issue and that you might want to use to help educate your children about additives in our food.

- "How It's Made Jawbreakers:" http://www.youtube.com/watch?v=NAgeGsFIRds. The video shows how much sugar and artificial food coloring (*paint*) go into the making of some popular candies.

- "Artificial Food Coloring and ADHD" (http://nutritionfacts.org/video/artificial-food-colors-and-adhd/)

- "Seeing Red No. 3: Coloring to Dye For" (http://nutritionfacts.org/video/seeing-red-no-3-coloring-to-dye-for/) by *NutritionFacts.org*.

Most of these food colorings are now banned in European countries. Amazingly, they've learned how to use natural food coloring instead (e.g. beets, turmeric, matcha, spirulina, spinach, blueberry, bentonite, coffee beans, etc.). So, global food companies (companies that sell in both Europe and the U.S.), sell one product in Europe and the lesser quality or product-with-unknown-and-potential-health risks is still marketed and sold in the U.S. Go figure!

Food Additives/Preservatives:

WARNING—this will probably make you feel like you are in a chemistry class, but you'll want to listen closely because I can almost guarantee that one, if not more, of these additives was in something that either you or your family ate today. Remember, studies are never conducted on humans AND of course they have never studied the effect of more than one of these "additives" in our food supply (or better yet our body) at the same time; they just wait to see what damage is done. SO, I guess you could say we are the lab rats!

- **Folic Acid** – is a man-made (synthetic) version of a critical B-vitamin (folate, vitamin B9). Our bodies are able to break down naturally-occurring folate from food (Dihydrofolate), but it takes many more steps and is much harder for our bodies to break down folic acid. As much as 50% of the population has genes that further slow the breakdown of folic acid.[xlvi]

  Deficiency in folate (the end-product of the vitamin breakdown) was found to cause neural tube defects in developing embryos. In an effort to decrease neural tube defects, the U.S. began adding folic acid to the food supply (all fortified flours, breads, pastries, cereals, pastas, even many drinks). Since that time, neural tube defects have in fact decreased. However, a whole host of DNA and brain problems have become more prominent (called methylation defects), especially among people who have great difficulty breaking down the synthetic form of this vitamin. Research has shown that we have just traded one problem for another by trying to mass-introduce this synthetic vitamin.

47

Methylation complications have been seen in mental disabilities, immune deficiency, cancer, atherosclerosis, dementia, increased aging and other diseases.[xlvii,xlviii,xlix] So, while a few pregnancy complications have been averted, what's been the cost? If you are someone who has a decreased ability to break down synthetic folic acid, the only way to prevent methylation complications is to completely avoid *all folic acid fortification* and to obtain your folate naturally through food (e.g. green leafy vegetables, fruit, nuts, beans, peas, meat, eggs, seafood, grains and more) and/or methyl-folate supplementation (always consult with a qualified doctor before adding supplements).

- **Tertiary Butylhydroquinone (TBHQ)** – is a chemical preservative which is a form of butane. It is commonly used in crackers, peanut butter, ramen noodles, fast foods including a popular type of chicken nugget, pet foods, cosmetic and baby skincare products, varnish, lacquers and resins. It is used to extend the shelf life of oily and fatty foods. The FDA allows amounts of up to 0.02% of the total oils in food to be TBHQ. There are questions as to whether it contributes to ADD/ADHD, asthma, rhinitis and dermatitis in humans and it has been shown to cause DNA damage and cancer in lab animals.[l]

- **Butylated hydroxyanisole (BHA)** – is a chemical preservative that is commonly found in potato chips, lard, butter, cereal, instant mashed potatoes, preserved meat, beer, baked goods, dry beverage and dessert mixes, chewing gum, rubber, petroleum products, and wax food packaging. It also keeps oily and fatty foods from going rancid on the shelf. While the FDA deems it to be "generally recognized as safe," the National Institute of Health says it's "reasonably anticipated to be a human carcinogen." Hmm…there's government consistency for you!

- **Butylated hydroxytoluene (BHT)** – is a chemical preservative, a derivative of phenol, which is used to preserve food odor, color, and flavor. Many packaging materials incorporate BHT. It is also added directly to shortening, cereals, and other foods containing fats and oils. While allowable by the FDA in small amounts, there is evidence that certain persons may have difficulty metabolizing both BHA and BHT, resulting in health and behavior changes.[li,lii]

- **Monosodium glutamate (MSG)** – is a flavor enhancer added to thousands of foods that your family may eat, especially if you eat fast food or in restaurants regularly. MSG is considered by many to be one of the worst food additives on the market. It is an excitotoxin, which means it overexcites your cells to the point of damage or death, causing brain damage to varying degrees, and potentially even triggering or worsening learning disabilities. Potential adverse effects of regular consumption of MSG include: obesity, eye damage, headaches, fatigue and disorientation, depression, rapid heartbeat, tingling and numbness.[liii,liv,lv]

- **Carrageenan** – is a common thickener (also gelling and stabilizing) used in hot/cold cocoa mixes, powdered milk, nutritional shakes, yogurt, non-dairy milk alternatives (e.g. almond milk, coconut milk, rice milk) and more. It's derived from red seaweed and has controversially been used even in many organic products. Carrageenan appears to be particularly destructive to the digestive system, triggering an immune response similar to one your body has when invaded by pathogens like Salmonella.[lvi,lvii] It appears that all food related irritations cause inflammation and *remember*, inflammation is at the root of most disease.

- **Xanthan Gum** – is a sugar-like compound made by mixing fermented sugars with a certain kind of bacteria. In medicine it is used as a laxative and for lowering blood sugar and total cholesterol in diabetics. In manufacturing, it is used as a common thickener and stabilization agent in foods, toothpastes and medicines. Xanthan Gum is strictly prohibited at the neo-natal departments; they were previously adding Xanthan Gum to the tube feeding for preemies, and it was creating holes in the intestines of the infants.[lviii,lix] **It has been advised that no one under the age of 12 months ingest Xanthan Gum**. Adverse symptoms in those over 12 months can include nausea, vomiting, appendicitis, hard stools that are difficult to expel (fecal impaction), narrowing or blockage of the intestine, or undiagnosed stomach pain. It appears that these reactions might be from the "sugar-like compound" used to make Xanthan Gum as it is often a potentially allergenic (or even GMO) substance such as corn, soy, dairy, or wheat.

Unintended additives: while food colorings are put there to increase food appeal and additives are there to enhance a food, there are other things that end up in foods that were never intended and can be quite harmful.

- **Xenoestrogens** – are a type of endocrine disruptor found in cosmetics, plastic food containers, plastic water bottles and more. Endocrine disruptors are a category of chemicals that alter the normal function of hormones. When chemicals from the outside get into our bodies, they have the ability to mimic our natural hormones; blocking or binding hormone receptors. This is particularly detrimental to hormone sensitive organs like the uterus and the breast, the immune and neurological systems, as well as human development. When xenoestrogens enter the body they increase the total amount of estrogen resulting in a phenomenon called, estrogen dominance. Xenoestrogens are not biodegradable so they are stored in our fat cells. Buildup of xenoestrogens have been indicated in many conditions including: breast, prostate and testicular cancer, obesity, infertility, endometriosis, early onset puberty, miscarriages and diabetes. As a final warning, **please do not EVER cook food in a plastic container in microwaves, drink water from a water bottle that has been heated by the sun (or left in a hot car), or put warm food or drinks in a plastic container (e.g. plastic mugs or putting a plastic straw into** a hot liquid), as this expedites the passage of the **xenoestrogens into your food and/or drink**.

- **Styrofoam containers** – are most often used for disposable (convenience) food packaging and take-out. Styrofoam is actually a brand name for the material, polystyrene (PS). It is denoted by a #6 or PS in the triangle on the bottom of food packaging. The single-molecule form of polystyrene is known as styrene. PS foam, the type used in food packaging for products like take-away containers, supermarket meat trays, etc., is created by injecting the plastic polymer, polystyrene, with a gas-such as HCFC 22, CFC 11, or CFC 12 (all ozone destroying chlorofluorocarbons), or pentane-to expand it into that puffy material. Toxic and hazardous chemicals, including styrene, benzene and ethylene, are used to make PS foam and are a byproduct of PS foam production. A 1988 survey published by the Foundation for Advancements in Science and Education also found styrene in human fatty tissue with a frequency of 100% at levels from 8 to 350 nanograms/gram (ng/g). The 350 ng/g level is one-third of levels known to cause neurotoxic symptoms. If you drink water, tea, or coffee from polystyrene cups four times a day for three years, you may have consumed about one Styrofoam cup-worth of styrene along with your beverages. Once styrene gets into your food or drink—and then into you—what does it do? Studies suggest that styrene mimics estrogens in the body and can therefore disrupt normal hormone functions, possibly contributing to thyroid problems, menstrual irregularities, and other hormone-related problems, as well as breast cancer and prostate cancer.[ix] Styrene is considered a possible human carcinogen by the World Health Organization's International Agency for Research on Cancer. So why, I ask, is Styrofoam still used on school campuses daily?

- **Foil, Non-Stick Pans and heavy metals in food** – People can be exposed to these metals from the environment or by ingesting contaminated food or water (contamination can occur during food processing and storage). Common sources of food contamination with metals include using foil to store and cook food, non-stick and aluminum pans to cook and prepared canned foods. Aluminum and lead have been linked to behavioral problems, learning disabilities, dementia and Alzheimer's. All metals can accumulate in the body and aluminum tends to travel to your brain and accumulate there.

It is important to note that for all food coloring and additives discussed here, there are research reports that will say they are "safe" to a certain level of consumption. What is critical is to see who *funded* those studies. When profits are at risk, corporations have been known to commission reports or studies that would find favor in their product. Our intuitive nature should be to question all such "studies" that are commissioned, paid for by or have the involvement of executives from companies who stand to make a profit.

We, you and I, and our children, are the new animals being used for testing! In 10-20 years when they find "problems" with the chemicals being used in our foods they will say "oops" and move on to the next chemical that hasn't been researched yet. I say, "STOP! Not with my family you won't!"

If there is no health benefit, but there is a potential risk, why does the government allow these substances into our food supply?

The only way to reduce the amount of chemicals, metals, hormone disruptors and potential carcinogens from your food is to read labels and eat whole foods (not coming from a package), at home, as often as is possible.

---

xlvi http://ajcn.nutrition.org/content/100/2/593.full; available September 19,

2014.

xlvii Costello, JF and Plass C. Methylation matters. *Journal of Medical Genetics*, 2001;38:285-303.

xlviii Robertson, K. DNA methylation and human disease. *Nature Reviews Genetics* 2005;6:597-610.

xlix Tost, J. DNA methylation: an introduction to the biology and the disease-associated changes of a promising biomarker. *Methods Mol Biol*. 2009;507:3-20

l Tert-Butylhydroquinone - safety summary from The International Programme on Chemical Safety
http://www.inchem.org/documents/jecfa/jecmono/v35je03.htm; available July 11, 2014.

li Gudz T et al. Effect of butylhydroxytoluene and related compounds on permeability of the inner mitochondrial membrane. Arch Biochem Biophys 1997 Jun 1;342(1):143-56.

lii Peters MM et al. Glutathione conjugates of tert-butyl-hydroquinone, a metabolite of the urinary tract tumor promoter 3-tert-butyl-hydroxyanisole, are toxic to kidney and bladder. *Jrnl of Cancer Research*:
http://cancerres.aacrjournals.org/content/56/5/1006.abstract ; available July 11, 2014.

liii http://articles.mercola.com/sites/articles/archive/2009/04/21/msg-is-this-silent-killer-lurking-in-your-kitchen-cabinets.aspx; available July 14, 2014.

liv Understanding brain damage and endocrine disorders caused by MSG, http://www.truthinlabeling.org/Dang.html

lv U.S. Food and Drug Administration "FDA and Monosodium Glutamate (MSG)" August 31, 1995.

lvi The International Agency for Research on Cancer of the World Health Organization classifies degraded carrageenan as a List 2B "possible human carcinogen."

lvii Tobacman JK (2001) Review of Harmful Gastrointestinal Effects of Carrageenan in Animal Experiments. Environmental Health Perspectives 109(10).

lviii Beal J, et al. Late onset necrotizing enterocolitis in infants following use of a xanthan gum-containing thickening agent. J Pediatr. 2012 Aug;161(2):354-6.

lix Woods CW, et al. Development of necrotizing enterocolitis in premature infants receiving thickened feeds using SimplyThick®. J Perinatol. 2012 Feb;32(2):150-2.

lx "Polystyrene Fact Sheet," Foundation for Advancements in Science and Education, Los Angeles, California.

PART II

FOOD AND LIFESTYLE HABITS ON CAMPUSES THAT PROMOTE DISEASE

We've learned that what we eat truly matters. We *are* what we eat! So, let's look at the typical "day" in the life of a typical American student:

Breakfast (if any):
boxed cereal with milk, egg sandwich, pastry or cup of yogurt

"Brunch" Break (common on many middle/high schools):
sports drink, breadsticks, cookies

School Lunch:
pizza, sloppy joe, hot dog or some sort of sandwich ... and milk

Afterschool Snack:
slice of pizza, chips, maybe another sports drink

Dinner:
possibly chicken or meat with veggies (one could hope!), spaghetti (or other pasta), pizza, hamburger or other fast food

WHERE, oh where, are the fruits and vegetables and whole (unprocessed) grains in these choices? The building blocks of lifetime health begin in infancy and continue through adolescence (and beyond). Yes, a school lunch may often be accompanied by a slice of fruit, but honestly, it is no wonder that obesity, high blood pressure and other diseases are on the rise in children. Their bodies cannot survive long on these food-like substances. If we want our children to outlive us and have quality, healthy lives, we *must* make a change now!

And, while school cafeterias limit the intake of oils and total calories in food served, they do *not* limit the amount of sugar. The sugar chapter in the previous section discusses how sugar is harmful to our bodies and plays a critical role in almost all diseases as well as with classroom focus, attention, behavior and performance (or lack thereof).

In 2013, 30.6 million children ate school lunch each day. School breakfast, which has experienced a 55.9% increase over the last decade, helps to ensure over 13.1 million children "have a healthy start" to their school day. Add it all up, and it's over 7 billion meals over the course of a school year. It's imperative that we ensure that those meals are nutritious, safe, and delicious for kids who are developing eating habits that will last a lifetime.

But as you can see from the title, we're not just going to be talking about food on school campuses, we're also going to be talking about the environment of school campuses (attitudes of staff regarding healthy food and lifestyle, modeling of healthy behavior, amount of time spent sitting, PE classes, bullying and more). And even the food…does it all come from just the cafeteria? No way! There is "food" in the classroom, vending machines on campus and sometimes even "snack bars" are available for students to purchase food-like-substances.

I thought it was important for you to be able to take a look at this following section through the eyes of a student, someone exposed to the environment today (which may or may not be what it was like when you and I were in school). I wish we could sit and talk with thousands of students across North America, get feedback and from it make meaningful change. I asked my son, Kelson, to write a portion for each of the chapters in this section. I hope you enjoy hearing what he had to say as much as I did.

CHAPTER 8

VENDING MACHINES AND SNACK BARS

Kelson, high school student:

Vending machines on school campuses are often a quick and easy way to get a bottle of water, or more likely, a bottle of a sugar-packed sports drink.

Often, during a "brunch" and/or lunch break, schools will also offer snacks for sale, such as a slice of pizza or a rice krispy treat in a small, either portable or permanent, snack bar.

In elementary school years it is unlikely you'll find a vending machine on the campus for general use—most likely because they don't expect kids that young to be carrying pocket change—but as you rise through the grades you'll find vending machines becoming more and more prevalent. After advancing from elementary school to middle school, you begin to see vending machines scattered across the campus containing sports drinks and water.

Usually the majority of the options are for a variety of sports drinks or juice-like products and then they leave one meager option at the very bottom for those searching for a bottle of water.

Children in middle school see these machines and instantly become filled with excitement at these beacons of freedom and choice. No longer do you have a parent or adult standing over you advising your choices. Here you can select whatever you'd like assuming you have the required dollar or two. It's not uncommon to witness a middle schooler or high schooler walk into class carrying a Gatorade or PowerAde, or maybe even two. Although teachers discourage these drinks in class (to avoid sticky messes of course, not out of any health concerns) it doesn't take much to slip one or two into your backpack and sneak a sip whenever the teacher has his or her back turned.

Snack bars provide the same freedoms, with the exception that you can now choose from food in addition to a drink. Snack bars typically provide small substitute lunch foods for kids who aren't looking for a full meal from the cafeteria, or who just find themselves having a grumbling tummy or craving and are looking for a quick fix. There's lots of wonderful choices (through a kid's eyes, anyway) to choose from including slices of pizza, Chinese fast food, salads, and the sort (although the salads might not be best placed under "wonderful choices" if you ask your average teen or preteen).

Vending machines and snack bars, in their current form, are quick ways for your child to access the less than desirable foods you may try to steer them away from at home.

Among the sugary and less healthy options, you could buy a cookie, a rice krispy treat, or even a bag of potato chips. Even if you don't limit their food options at home, they now have the ability to spend the money for lunch that you gave them on other things, such as several cookies instead of a lunch.

Dr. Angela:

For the past five or so years, many campuses have been consciously removing soda from their school's vending machines, due to the widespread understanding and numerous studies showing the harms of heavy soda consumption during childhood. Believe me, there was quite a grumble from schools as these vending machines are a source of revenue to them. And, whether the school administration knew it or not, Pepsi and Coke simply replaced their sugar-laden sodas with sugar-laden "sports" and "energy" drinks. Full Throttle and NOS (energy drinks) and PowerAde (sports drink) are Coca Cola, while Moutain Dew KickStart (energy drink) and Gatorade (sports drink) are Pepsi branded drinks that contain as much if not more sugar than their sodas did, but are "technically" now allowed on school campuses in their place. Of course the energy drinks are also enhanced with caffeine and/or other stimulants.

If your local campuses have not removed or at least greatly reduced their on-campus vending machines, this is a good thing to start with. What the vending machines contain *in* them is an even larger issue that needs to be resolved. Water alone should be enough for our students throughout the day and they shouldn't have to consult with a money-making machine to gain access to clean, filtered drinking water!

FOOD FOR THOUGHT:

How are you going to discuss this "temptation," its health implications and alternative solutions with your child?

CHAPTER 9

CAFETERIAS

Kelson, high school student:

Much like the snack bars, your typical school cafeteria will contain a large variety of foods for children to choose from. Here, instead, you'll find more foods that you could reasonably call a lunch. There's sandwiches, hamburgers, more pizza, salads, and so on. Here most of the options you buy come with a drink and a side.

You'd think that the dairy companies ran the schools the way the younger grade levels shove milk down your throat, offering only regular milk, chocolate milk, and occasionally strawberry milk as the drink options. If you had any desire to have a bottle of water instead of the incredibly processed and preserved milk of another animal, you could slip the lunch lady an extra dollar* and receive a bottle of water in return, which makes life incredibly difficult (and more costly) for someone with dairy allergies such as myself. However, in high school they seem to have realized that forcing milk on every student might not be the greatest financial venture, and instead offer it for free with your meal.

When it comes to the sides offered with a cafeteria lunch, they vary with grade level, in that as you go up in grade level so do the calories of the sides offered. In elementary school students will be given an apple or kiwi, something relatively healthy if you ignore the preservatives and pesticides they're likely covered in. Middle Schools begin to offer salads on top of fruit, but more importantly (to the kids, that is) they begin to offer bags of potato chips or French fries as a side. You can also request a cookie if you have a couple extra quarters to throw around.

I've always taken precautions to avoid the cafeterias of my schools even before I was conscious about my allergies, as the food they provide is generally twice frozen over and just plain disgusting. Even now in high school I see some of the "meals" my friends bring out of the cafeteria, and the fat and grease is more visible than any of the ingredients in the food. A close friend of mine is forced to buy and eat school food, but even he scoffs at it before eating, and eats without any pleasure in doing so. He once ordered a salad, and opened it up for us to see the layer of pure fat over all the chicken inside the salad.

With my allergies school food is just completely out of the picture (one might almost call it a perk of having said allergies), as they don't offer a single option that doesn't contain either dairy or gluten inside it. Even the salads are smothered in ranch dressing.

I escaped elementary school before they started distributing "breakfast" directly in the classroom. It would have even been harder yet at such a young age—it's a sugarholic's dream—but absolutely off-the-hook for somebody with my allergies: sugared breakfast cereals, pancakes and such, of course, served up with milk.

*When Kelson was in Elementary school, water was not an alternative option at lunch and he had to pay extra for it.

Dr. Angela:

Some parents might read Kelson's description in this chapter and think, "I'll just send lunch to school with my child." I hope that continues to be an option. In some schools, parents are being told that they are not allowed to send food from home (without a doctor's note)![lxi] On April 11, 2011, the *Chicago Tribune* reported that Chicago schools banned foods from home.[lxii]

In other schools, where a parent chose to send lunch to school with their child, the school has taken it upon themselves to "supplement" the child's lunch and *charge the parents* for said service. Note: Ritz crackers were provided as the child had what was deemed to be a "grain-free" lunch.[lxiii] According to the nutrition facts found on its homepage, a serving of Ritz crackers (~10 crackers) contains 6.5g of fat, of which nearly half is saturated. And never mind that the school's idea of "grain" is a processed, packaged, calorie-laden and nutrition-barren Frankenstein-food-like-substance!

According to Weighty Matters, the Manitoba Government's Early Learning and Child Care department blindly follows a policy which requires lunches to be "balanced according to Canada's awful Food Guide." Unbalanced lunches are subject to supplementation and a fine of CDN$5 (US$4.80) per "missing item" per child. To drive home the ridiculousness of the policy, a mom told Weighty Matters she could have sent her kids to daycare with "microwave Kraft Dinner and a hot dog, a package of fruit twists, a string cheese, and a juice box," and it would have been met with approval by the MCCA.

In my opinion, the government has *not* done a good job of educating its citizens about food health, maintaining government food guidelines that are based on current nutritional research or implementing school food programs that are nutritious and healthy. So *why* are they usurping parents' rights to do so?

FOOD FOR THOUGHT:

How are you going to ensure that your child is free from food allergens and is able to eat nutritious food while at school?

[lxi] Momdot Blog, "What the Wha??" http://www.momdot.com/a-doctors-note-for-gmos/; available 7/17/14.

[lxii] http://articles.chicagotribune.com/2011-04-11/news/ct-met-school-lunch-

restrictions-041120110410_1_lunch-food-provider-public-school; available 1/23/14.

[lxiii] Momables Blog, Mom Gives Kid Homemade Lunch, School Forces Kid to Eat Crackers. http://www.momables.com/mom-gives-kid-homemade-lunch-school-forces-kid-to-eat-crackers/; available 7/17/14.

CHAPTER 10

PEER AND CLASSROOM ENVIRONMENT

Dr. Angela on Sugar in Elementary School Classrooms:

There is a video available on *YouTube*, "How to Magnetize a Baby,"[lxiv] that shows a social experiment using sugar to magnetize a baby, elicit pleasure and a positive response to the person providing the sugar.

As with sugar and babies' responses to the generous donor, so it goes in elementary school. Although many teachers are no longer "supposed to" (various districts have passed policies disallowing food as incentives), they still often use various forms of sugar in the classroom as incentives or rewards. Also, when it is a child's birthday or there is a holiday to celebrate, it seems as if the Class Parent and/or all other parents compete to see who can bring the most elaborate and sweetest confections.

Some of us may even see ourselves in this sentiment. I'm guilty! I took cupcakes to school for birthdays. And, let's face it, if this were the only sugar these kids consumed in a day, it might not be damaging. But with kids who have sugar addictions, kids who have insulin sensitivity, kids who have gluten and/or other allergies and/or sensitivities, that one cupcake or treat could be the thing that sets them off!

Remember, while school cafeterias may have a limit as to how much fat they are allowed to serve, there are no such regulations around sugar. By the time many kids leave elementary school, they have already been set up with sugar addictions, only to launch them into the chaos and peer pressure of middle (or Junior High) school.

Kelson, on being a teen in middle and high school:

Imagine yourself being a 6th or 7th grader, fresh out of elementary school and looking to make good with your peers in middle school. You may have been scolded and directed away from sugary candy or drinks at home, but there are no parents here. You walk into class and see the most popular kid wielding a bottle of Gatorade with another peeking out of his backpack. Obviously there's something cool about drinking Gatorade, right? No pressure though. It's not like you just entered some of the most socially awkward and difficult years of your life and are looking for ways to get people to like you or anything. (Translation: this is teenage sarcasm!)

Other kids can often provide the most pressure towards eating foods that you may not normally have an affinity for. I've seen kids bashed for what they eat at school, or for bringing a healthier option to a class party. Why be the person who brings carrots and hummus to the party when you can be the kid who brings three boxes of Oreos, right?

Sophomore year of high school I had a brutally honest but effective teacher who often said "Want some friends? Buy some cupcakes and hand them out." Nobody (except for maybe those one or two vegetarian or vegan girls) would feel a particular drive to make friends with a kid who brings broccoli and hands it out.

And although it's against the rules, kids also began buying large boxes of assorted candy and selling the individual candies for profit. It worked like a charm; the boxes sold out in a day or two. If you see someone walking around selling your favorite candy for a dollar in the middle of the day, there's a decent chance you'll go and buy said candy. These kids bring the stuff you can't purchase from the cafeteria and sell it for a meager dollar per bar/piece, which just gives kids another opportunity to access the sugar high they've been craving all day after sitting around twiddling their thumbs in a classroom.

In Closing

How do we reverse our programming? How do we "unlearn" the idea that a candy is a treat and to spoil a child is to take them out for a spectacular ice cream sundae? Why do we compete for our kids' affections using sugar? I call uncle! Let's reverse this trend. Let's learn to use other modes of positive rewards in the classroom ("book" time, earn points to win educational prizes, etc.) and let's learn, as parents, to support class parties in a healthier manner: fruit cakes (literally, a cake made from fruit – check them out on *YouTube*!), raw snacks, vegetables and dips, fruit smoothies—let's put our heads together and come up with an entire list. No more sugar addicted kids due to our affections (or our need to win it from them)!

FOOD FOR THOUGHT:

How are you going to support a healthier classroom environment in elementary school and/or help your child become pressure-proof— from sugar and many more substances (or "offers") that *will* be coming their way?

---

lxiv How to Magnetize a Baby, https://www.youtube.com/watch?v=bRFpLdv6LYk; available 7/23/14.

CHAPTER 11

"HEALTH" EDUCATION

Kelson:

In elementary school, there is supposedly a requirement placed on teachers to add so many hours of "health." I don't remember receiving any such instruction from a PE or classroom teacher. In middle school there was one semester (half a school year) dedicated to health education. The only thing I remember about it is—a positive—participating in the care and keeping (and eating from) the school garden. I still remember how great the cherry tomatoes tasted. We also covered some anti-smoking and drug awareness stuff. We had a project about bullying, but it just made me realize that the adults had no idea how the insidious bullying happens today.

In high school, there is a mandatory class that, in theory, should teach you how to take care of your body to ensure a healthy, happy life. **Health education classes can be summarized in three points: don't have sex, don't drink or do drugs, and eat healthy.**

Unfortunately they don't exactly teach you *how* to eat healthy. The class tends to focus on the first two, with a little section thrown in there for food. They teach you the basic food groups (on the much outdated food pyramid), that an excessive calorie intake is bad, and how to read nutrition labels. That's it.

There's so many more levels of nutrition education that people could use to make smart food choices. Eating more calories than your recommended daily amount can be bad for your body, **but there is a visible difference between the calories**

67

in fruits and vegetables than those in sugar and meat.

So, before middle school no official classes were set aside for health education, it was mostly just small short school assemblies and the occasional random lesson via a teacher looking out for you. Since these random efforts and even formal classes fail to give you all the information you need to make great food choices, **the only direction towards healthy choices you get might be that given to you from your parents.** School may be a great place to learn "reading, writing and arithmetic," but perhaps not the best place to learn how to lead a healthy and happy life (at least not yet).

Even my peers don't discuss food in terms of nutrition much while at school. It's more about taste: "yum" or "yuck." Like I said, not much enjoyment around food on campus. I guess I've stirred up more conversations around food than is normal because people tend to notice when I avoid what everyone else is eating. They generally ask why and I've begun to educate them in small ways. But I don't feel like an expert on the matter. I feel like some adult should be filling in the blanks: why are so many kids reacting to gluten, having issues with weight, getting diagnosed with autism, ADD and other diseases? What gives? Why does it feel like we're an afterthought?

Dr. Angela:

The Food Guide Pyramid that Kelson referred to is part of the historical USDA *Dietary Guidelines for Americans.*[lxv]

The *Food Pyramid*, still being used in many public schools today, is out of date and scientifically inaccurate.

It was originally incorporated by the USDA in 1992, updated in 2005 (adding "oils" and a discussion about exercise) and was replaced by *MyPyramid* in 2010. The USDA was successfully sued and lost (unprecedented) for *MyPyramid* as it was not consistent with scientific research. The current model, *MyPlate*, is again under attack as the USDA continues to cave to lobby pressures rather than following independent scientific research. The *Dietary Guidelines for Americans* are supposed to be reviewed every five years and are up for review again in 2015.

Most schools continue to also promote the "exercise more and eat less" philosophy for health and weight loss. At a total-caloric-intake level this may seem reasonable, but where it fails is in understanding the quality of each calorie and how food talks to our hormones. As Kelson said above, fruits and vegetables speak one language (to our body), meat another, and sugar yet another entirely. A calorie is not a calorie!

Everything that we eat and drink translates into chemical and hormonal messages to our cells, hormones, and ultimately our organs, including our brain. If we want our children to avoid ADD/ADHD, obesity, metabolic syndrome, depression, heart disease, cancers, autoimmune conditions and more, we ***must*** start having a conversation about the quality of foods and what messages we are sending to our bodies!

Many who are teaching the required health classes received their education some years prior and most likely also received outdated information at that time. There is no requirement for ongoing education for teachers who impart this information to our students. Many may also *not* be good role models themselves. Finally, there are not a lot of strict standards for curriculum used (much of it comes from or is subsidized by various "industries") and course standards may or may not be set and enforced by districts.

Nutrition is *the* fastest growing field of science today.

If schools can't keep up (apparently even the USDA can't keep up), why are we expecting them to be able to educate our children on this topic? So, if parents are to be relied upon as being the first and most important resource on this topic, we have some work to do! We also received well-meaning but inaccurate information during our own school education and have been programmed by advertising and marketing from all of the various "industries." So, where are you going to get sufficient education to bolster your children's health?

Kelson and I would be honored to be a partner in your quest. It is our hope that the content you find in this book motivates you to keep learning. There will be additional resources available at http://www.AngelaGriffithsDC.com/HealtheChildren. We absolutely encourage you to communicate with us through the site and let us know if there are additional topics that we can provide research on in order to help you make the best decisions for your family!

FOOD FOR THOUGHT:

What steps are you going to take to better educate yourself, and then your child, about nutrition in general and on what food should regularly be on your plate?

[lxv] A Brief History of USDA Food Guides http://www.choosemyplate.gov/food-groups/downloads/MyPlate/ABriefHistoryOfUSDAFoodGuides.pdf; available July 23, 2014.

CHAPTER 12

NUMBER OF HOURS SITTING

Kelson:

There's not much excitement in your average classroom. It's not as if you're getting up and running around constantly; quite the opposite actually. It's up to two hours every class, seven hours per day, with the exception of a brief passing period between classes, a 10-minute break early in the day and a 45-minute lunch break. So, you ask, *where* did we learn to become couch potatoes? Okay, no couches at school, but still.

In my high school we use a "block schedule" that makes classes on Tuesdays and Wednesdays two hours long, although you only have three classes in a day. Even with fewer classes, sitting for two hours straight can be plain torture. After sophomore year you no longer have to take physical education as a class either, so there can be literally zero physical activity in the school day.

Most students also find a desirable spot to place themselves down for lunch and then don't move for the rest of the period, so even during that break from the forced seating, the majority of kids don't choose to move around. The lack of exercise or movement can leave kids feeling bored and unengaged, and result in seven hours of an almost completely sedentary day. (That's not even to mention what my generation tends to do when we get home.)

Dr. Angela:

Dr. Len Kravitz, an exercise scientist, talks about how sitting has become a disease. He, along with many other specialists, states that decreases in our daily movement (called Non-Exercise Activated

Thermogenesis or NEAT) cause changes in energy balance and may be important in the physiology of weight change. In other words, it's not just the one hour of exercise in PE or at the gym, it's the repetitive small movements throughout the day that make a difference for our weight and health.[lxvi,lxvii, lxviii,lxix]

> *Sitting was once a break in a busy day. Now it is the singular way most of us spend our time. Take a moment to reflect on a typical day. How did you get to work? Like 98% of Americans, you probably either drove or sat on a bus, train, or subway car. If you work in an office, the rest of your day was likely spent chairbound—at your desk, in endless meetings, or having lunch. What do you do after work? Sit down at the computer to pay some bills, shop online, catch up on e-mail? And after that? Maybe kick back and unwind with a few of your favorite shows?* James A. Levine, MD, PhD *Move a Little, Lose a Lot*

While schools have been putting an increased emphasis on academics, they seem not to put much importance into the amount of time students spend moving during the day. In Dr. Carla Hannaford's book, *Smart Moves: Why Learning Is Not All In Your Head*, she states that bodily movements and brain growth and health (the ability to think and learn) are intimately connected. Movement is also connected with balance, gross motor skills, sensory perception in our nerves, vision, digestion, and much, much more. There are many more scientists and articles that substantiate the points she is making. Why then do schools keep our kids sedentary for so long? We need to help them get moving, for the sake of their health, their intelligence and their lives!

A source for ideas to help get kids and families moving comes from www.letsmove.gov: walk to work, walk during your lunch hour, walk instead of driving whenever you can, take a family walk after dinner, skate to work instead of drive, mow the lawn with a push mower, walk your dog, work and walk around the house, wash the car by hand, bike with family and friends, perform gardening and/or home repairs, **avoid sitting for more than 30-minutes at a time**, play with your kids 30-minutes a day, dance to music, walk briskly in the mall, take the stairs instead of the escalator, go for a hike.

NOTE: (another government inconsistency) they recommend not sitting for more than 30-minutes at a time but allow schools to create schedules that allow students to sit for up to two-hours or more at a time.

FOOD FOR THOUGHT:

What's one small change that you and your child can make to increase your daily amount of movement (small movements throughout your entire day)?

[lxvi] Kravitz, L. (2009). Too much sitting is hazardous to your health. IDEA Fitness Journal, 6(9), 14-17.

[lxvii] Kravitz, L. (2006). A NEAT "new" strategy for weight control. IDEA Fitness Journal, 3(4), 24-25.

[lxviii] Levine, James A. Move a Little Lose a Lot. Three Rivers Press, 2009.

[lxix] Katzmarzyk, PT et al. (2009). Sitting time and mortality from all causes, cardiovascular disease, and cancer. Medicine & Science in Sports & Exercise, 41(5),998-1005.

CHAPTER 13

PHYSICAL EDUCATION (PE)

Kelson on "PE in School":

I was lucky. In elementary school, we got to have PE a couple times per week (many other schools have already cut this out). We actually had a very energetic teacher who was a true role model. The days that we didn't have PE were just kind of random chaos on the playground, which I didn't mind so much, but I would see other kids sitting on the side of the playground reading or otherwise just trying to make themselves invisible.

In middle and high school, PE as a class can either be a joke or a very dreadful thing. Being forced to change in the middle of the day and drench yourself in sweat can be horrid, but on the other hand a large number of PE teachers manage to get away without working their students at all. Since middle school I've experienced a few of each type of PE teachers and classes.

One such teacher had a physical appearance to match his work ethic: slow and lazy. It's criminal that they would allow someone to order a student to do something that the teacher themselves couldn't do.

A math teacher can perform any equation they give to a student, so why can't some PE teachers perform the tasks they assign their students?

Some PE teachers also seem to have realized this and so instead of becoming a better role model they simply assign their students what they can do: nothing. Every day I was given the offhand order to walk a lap around the track, and then loiter around until the bell rang. It provided an hour to two hours a day of doing literally nothing except socializing with my friends. Personally I don't have any complaints about doing so, although I will willingly admit that it has no place in the school day.

On the other hand, my second year of high school provided me with a PE teacher of quite the opposite nature. This one could not only do what he assigned for us to do he could run laps around us while doing it. Along with the change of role model came a change of pace, naturally. In his class you could expect to be covered in sweat by the end of the class period, assuming you did what he told you to. It was a rewarding feeling, working so hard to better my body, but it also came with the disgusting feeling of being drenched in sweat in the middle of a school day. I mean even though you're able to change your clothes, you still carry the sweat and smell with you … and that gross after-exercise hair.

Dr. Angela (with input from her project staff from the fitness and nutrition grant):

Physical activity is diminishing on school campuses.

- Kids spend 5-7 hours of sitting (aside from the time they spend in PE).

- There is decreased PE in elementary levels due to budget cuts and/or a lack of priority by the school districts.

- There are rising class sizes in middle and high school that make it difficult for PE teachers to keep all students engaged, learning and moving.

75

- Different PE teachers engage, encourage and expect varying outcomes from their students.

While fitness is recognized as an important component in health (especially in light of today's obesity and diabetes epidemics and the programs to mitigate those epidemics, such as the Let's Move campaign), the way it is "standardized" and applied in schools through physical education is not conducive to real and sustainable change.

Each state has physical education program standards. However, these standards are more recommendations than anything else. At the elementary level, very little reporting is required. In fact, many districts do not have assessment standards for the elementary level. And many districts are indeed halting formal physical education for elementary students, expecting classroom teachers to know how (and want to) pick up the slack.

Lack of fitness seems not to be as big of a concern at the Elementary level, as many kids play of their own accord and enjoy activity. The pitfall of this is that kids that are at-risk may not be caught early enough, important stability and balance skills may not be taught and the ability to track lifetime fitness is lost without the start of early measurement.

When students enter middle school, more reporting is required on their physical fitness levels and the students are required to achieve a level of fitness in order to pass their physical education class. Once again, this presents a pitfall that this can be especially difficult for students who are not able to achieve this age- and gender-specific standard as they have never had to meet a standard before and therefore are unprepared (e.g. timed mile, numbers of push-ups, etc.). Assessment is generally required at an interval such as in the 5th, 7th and 9th grades, during which time a student's physical fitness level can change significantly.

Students will face similar standards in high school; however, they will only have to do so through their sophomore year (only two years of physical education is required). Thereafter, their physical activity and fitness levels will be determined solely on their own accord. This usually occurs in the form of sports, so a large portion of students will not be physically active, as many do not have the proclivity towards, financial means for or interest in sports.

Students need to learn fitness skills that they will be able to use and modify over the course of their lifetime.

Another issue with the standards set by a state is that most are team-sport focused. While this is not without merit as it can be beneficial for students to learn about strategy and team work, it makes up the bulk of the standards. This is problematic for two reasons: 1) it alienates students who may not be compatible with team sports and 2) it is generally not sustainable as most athletes cannot and will not be able to play the sport of their choice over a lifetime.

The next issue that arises with physical education standards is that Common Core (academic standards) is a major focus across school districts. America has been falling behind academically for several years and as a result the "unnecessary" subjects have been whittled away: PE and the arts. This has occurred despite the fact that America is also battling an obesity epidemic and that several studies report the benefits of physical activity on academic performance. This is not to say that physical education is more important than academics, but it should be treated as equally important as we have reached the point where many parents are expected to outlive their children.

During times of financial crisis, PE is one of the first subjects to have its budget cut.

Many districts face funding cuts and, because PE is generally considered a non-academic subject, it usually results in greater cuts. These cuts have often resulted in larger class sizes, which can make it difficult to effectively teach fitness concepts, keep all students moving, and becomes a safety issue.

Another potential consequence of funding cuts is fewer qualified teachers. Teachers who are tenured may be forced to teach physical education classes, though that may not be their specialty because the district cannot afford physical education teachers. Lack of funding also jeopardizes the continuing education of physical education teachers, since in these conditions they have to pay out of their own pockets to attend conferences and trainings. Furthermore, lack of funding affects a more basic need to purchase new or replace old equipment.

After spending the last three years working with students and collecting assessments in public schools, with the aim of seeing greater physical activity in kids over time, what we saw was that kids who come from *families that move* tended to support and engage more with their family movement activities (tennis, bike riding, hiking, kayaking, etc.). Kids who come from families who did not *move as a family,* had no change. It was rather sad.

MY TAKEAWAY:

- Schools need to do everything in their power to get every child/adolescent up and moving every 30-40 minutes.

- Schools need to get every child/adolescent active and learning lifetime fitness skills in PE (from Kindergarten on).

- Adults in schools need to model and value these principles. If kids/adolescents do not have role models at home, they certainly need them at school.

- Parents need to *find the time* to move with their families: even if you are exhausted, consistency in this area will *give you more energy.*

FOOD FOR THOUGHT:

As an extension from the thought activity from the last chapter (daily small movements), what fitness skills can you learn and/or start doing together as a family?

CHAPTER 14

BULLYING

Kelson:

Bullying in school can easily affect how children eat—either how much or what. I've witnessed cases where kids are harassed for the food they bring to school, until they began to bring foods that they thought would ease the bullying. Or kids that are regularly called fat and so they choose to eat so little or nothing at all.

Bullying often occurs to someone who looks or does *anything* different than their peer group...including healthy eating.

Bullies are often insecure about something in themselves. For instance, if they don't eat healthy food, they often can't handle that other people do, so they tease them for *not* conforming to the average kid's terrible diet. In short, they even harass a kid for doing the *right* thing! When you're looking for approval from your peers you'll willingly change that which can be changed easily—your food.

Dr. Angela:

Bullying can come in any form and for any reason. And it can be quite serious, even leading to suicide for what might *seem* to be something minor or inconsequential. Being accepted, feeling included in a peer group has never been inconsequential to any of us.

We have all tried to "fit in" (whatever that might mean). And how each person interprets the bullying is quite different. But when you have a peer group that *witnesses* the bullying and does nothing to stop it you can be made to feel even further separation.

I think that most of us can remember a time when we were ourselves bullied. For me, it happened in middle school. I was "too tall," stuck out like a sore thumb (chased home with threats of being beaten up, chided across crowded campus corridors, and mocked in the campus paper). There was at least a year where I did not have one friend on my school campus. But it didn't follow me into high school because I learned to not care and to live my own life. I was fortunate – I had my spiritual faith, my best friend (who attended another school) and my family to push me, bolster me and make me stick through it and not give up or give in.

If you are doing something (anything!) different, someone may bully or coerce you into coming back into line. As someone who has not eaten the *Standard American Diet (SAD)* for over 25 years, I often find myself at a dining table with someone questioning my food choices or teasing/mocking me for not eating what they are eating. I study food for a living! Why would I want to eat like them? But, even though I know the research, I do not sit at a table, criticize others and tell them how they should eat … **What is this societal pressure of "bullying," used to force someone to comply with social will? It's B.S.! But it *IS real*.**

The CDC states that bullying is a type of "youth violence."[lxx] I contend that bullying exists also in adulthood. Heck, while in high school, I even had an adult coach bully me *in front of my peers*! I find that bullying is engrained in our political system (e.g. lobbying, the act of passing legislation, elections).

How are we to tell a child that bullying is *inappropriate* when they regularly see and hear adults doing it?

Adults on school campuses, on the television, across the Internet (don't get me started on the forums on *Facebook* and other e-bullying!) regularly bully other peers, coworkers and children. Quite often it's all done in the name of saying, "I am *right* and therefore you are *wrong.*" Whatever happened to respect for an individual's decisions or opinions? I think we, as adults, have failed to model this for quite some time.

So how **do** we help our children become bully-proof, that they might continue making the best decisions for their health, wearing clothes that are comfortable to them, and acting in ways that make them feel good about themselves? And how do we prevent our children from becoming the bullies (because often those who have been bullied later become the bullies themselves)?

From the time they are young:

- Teach your children to respect a person, even if he/she doesn't look like them, or doesn't agree with the thoughts, behaviors or actions of that person.

- Help your child begin to see life through the eyes of other people (e.g. what would it be like to live like that, to have those kind of parents, to have lost a parent, to live with a disability, etc.).

- Help your children understand the nature of a bully—someone who has deep insecurities of their own; people who are comfortable with themselves and loving of others do not feel the need to tear someone else down.

- Help your children learn to connect with their own spirituality – we all have it within us and it is a deeper and higher power that helps us survive rough and lonely experiences. A church, synagogue, temple, mosque, etc. is just a building and it is filled with religion. I am not saying religion is faith. Spirituality is a deep personal bond and connection with your higher power. Kids will have to find that connection personally if it is going to help them, but you can certainly help guide them to find their connection.

- Teach your child how to respond as a witness to bullying (e.g. intervene either publicly or privately, depending upon their comfort, maturity and safety; report it to an adult if uncomfortable personally intervening).

- Help your child, as the receiver, learn not to respond to bullying; the more they respond, the more the bullying continues. Teach your child how not to feel like a victim.

This is an open conversation. I don't have all the answers. I would *love* to hear how you have helped your children become bully-proof. I want to hear about the miraculous things they have overcome and how they are learning to thrive!

FOOD FOR THOUGHT:

Is there possibly a way in which you might model a bullying behavior in front of your child (regarding politics, a relative who annoys you, etc.)? How might you turn this behavior around and maybe even turn it into a teaching moment for your child? If not, it wouldn't be hard to look around and find societal examples. Ask your child, did you see any forms of bullying at school today? How did it make you feel to see or be a victim of that? I try to check in with my kids on this pretty regularly.

[lxx] Youth Bullying: What Does the Research Say?
http://www.cdc.gov/ViolencePrevention/youthviolence/bullyingresearch/;
available 7/25/14.

PART III

MOST COMMON DISEASES CAUSED BY FOOD AND LIFESTYLE

"Let food be thy medicine and medicine be thy food." – Hippocrates

Apparently, somewhere along our recent ancestral line (within the last 100 years), we forgot that what we consume is not *just* for enjoyment or convenience; it has always been about nourishing our bodies.

Food is not just calories; it is hormonal information to our cells.

From the time food enters our mouth, until we excrete the portions of it that our body could not use or is done with, we are receiving messages. We break down the macronutrient calories for energy, extract fiber to nourish our microbiota, and keep our bowel movements normal, while the micronutrients (antioxidants, phytonutrients, enzymes and more that research has not even learned about yet) keep our cells, nerves, brain and organs healthy!

This "unique synergy" is no longer in play in many people's bodies. When the information that our cells receive is primarily from man-made food-like-substances (e.g. everything but the macronutrients has been stripped out and sometimes synthetic versions of micronutrients are added back in, as in many grains and milk), our cells, and eventually our health, suffer.

Our primary food sources are no longer developed by nature and grown in the earth.

Unfortunately, many children today are eating their way to disease on school campuses (and in many homes) in North America. This is not just sad, it is criminal!

Childhood is the most important period in our lifetime for setting up our body for lifelong health or disease.

Most Western medical doctors did not have the benefit of learning about the unique beauty and benefit of nutrition during their formal training. Again, it is sad. Somehow, instead, Western medicine has decided that pharmaceutical agents are qualified to be the source of our health. However, no pills have ever truly reversed disease … they simple mute the symptoms, while often causing a host of other symptoms and allowing diseases to escalate.

Most of all chronic diseases of our day are caused, and can be cured, by food.

That's right. How we eat allows the diseases to set up shop in our bodies. Now, for some of us, that makes us really mad, because we have done our very best to provide nutritious foods to our bodies and our families. Unfortunately, the information provided to us by our government was not always stellar and did not have the highest standard of proof working in our favor.

Pharmaceutical, agricultural, and food industries have been allowed to add things to our food, to change the DNA and nature of our food (hybridize and genetically modify plants) and to spray toxic chemicals on the produce and animals that we consume. Most of this has been done without having to prove to the government that those products will *not cause* harm. No studies have ever been done on humans using genetically modified organisms (GMO). We were simply "told" that they would not hurt us.

Are we going to sit back and wait for a disease to be diagnosed before we stand up and demand change?

"I'm sorry to tell you, but your son has diabetes" or "your daughter has cancer." I don't know if this is acceptable to you, but it is *not* for me. If someone told you that you could optimize your child's genes so that *none* of these diseases have to be realized, what would you say? What would you be willing to do?

I'm not saying it's going to be easy. In fact, it will be rather counter-culture. Are you in? Is your child's health worth it? The following chapters are some of the many diseases that are in store for many of our families if we don't act soon. And finally, the last section will be some of the action steps that you can start taking today. I will be your partner!

CHAPTER 15

ATTENTION DEFICIT DISORDERS (ADD/ADHD)

Attention Deficit Disorders (ADD and ADHD), collectively referred to as ADD here, are characterized primarily by toxicity in the brain and body, which causes metabolic dysfunction. Also, simple deficiencies in brain nutrition, caused by our unhealthy and often toxic food supply, can contribute to the onset.[lxxi]

ADD has increased by at least 400% over the past 20 years.

Now, 3.5 million children suffer from it. The very worst symptoms of ADD are similar to those of children on the autism spectrum. American kids now consume 90% of the world's Ritalin, the most popular ADD medication. It is the most common learning and behavior problem in children. But the issue doesn't end there: It is also one of the most common problems in adults, and has been associated with job failures, relationship breakups, loneliness, a tremendous sense of underachievement, etc. Untreated ADD increases the risk of high school dropout, depression, drug abuse, obesity, smoking, Type 2 diabetes, and Alzheimer's disease.[lxxii]

For over 20 years, Dr. Daniel Amen has been conducting brain imaging studies to try and understand *why* ADD is increasing and what is at its root. Studies show that **diet and exercise can impact ADD**. In a replicated study from Europe, 70 percent of ADD children showed greater than a 50 percent reduction of symptoms on an elimination diet, which concluded that food intake can make ADD symptoms better or worse.

In another study, exercise significantly enhanced executive function in ADD children.[lxxiii] Dr. Amen contends that the reduction of PE in schools (which has most severely impacted the youngest of our children, as elementary schools are generally the first to lose PE programs) may be costing our society much more in the long run in terms of lost learning and productivity.

There Are Five Hallmark Symptoms of ADD:

- **Short attention span for regular, routine, everyday tasks.** People with ADD have a difficult time with boring tasks and need stimulation or excitement in order to stay engaged. Many people with ADD can pay attention just fine for things that are new, novel, interesting, highly stimulating, or frightening.

- **Distractibility.** People with ADD tend to notice more in their environment than others, which makes them easily distracted by outside stimuli, such as light, sounds, smells, certain tastes, or even the clothes they wear. Their keen sensitivity causes them to get easily off task.

- **Disorganization.** Most people with ADD tend to struggle with the organization of time and space. They tend to be late and have trouble completing tasks on time. Many things get done at the last moment or even later. They also tend to struggle keeping their spaces tidy, especially their rooms, book bags, filing cabinets, drawers, closets, and paperwork.

- **Procrastination.** Tasks and duties get put off until the last moment. Things tend not to get done until there are deadlines or someone else is mad at them for not doing it.

- **Poor internal supervision.** Many people with ADD have issues with judgment and impulse control, and struggle not to say or do things without fully thinking them through. They also have a harder time learning from their mistakes.

Something else that I learned from Dr. Amen, **"ADD is not one thing."** There are actually seven types of ADD and it is possible to have more than one type. He expresses that to know your type is essential for getting the right help to heal—and there are natural treatments for each subtype.

Dr. Natasha Campbell-McBride has studied how food affects mood in both children and adults and how the health of our gut affects our brain and psychology. Because ultimately, if your gut (digestive system) is not healthy, you are unable to absorb nutrients from your food (assuming you are feeding it quality nutrients to begin with) and therefore your brain and body are not getting what they need to support proper function of your hormones, neurotransmitters, detoxification pathways, etc.[lxxiv]

Yet another specialist in this area, Dr. Kenneth Bock, further explains that:

The epidemic of ADD (as well as autism, asthma and allergies) is caused primarily by four fundamental, catastrophic changes in the environments of American children.

1. **Toxins Proliferated** – air and water pollution, foods fouled with chemicals, hormones and antibiotics

2. **Nutrition Deteriorated** – declining intake of essential nutrients (unrefined carbohydrates, protein, essential fatty acids, vitamins, minerals, enzymes, fiber, phytonutrients and antioxidants), increased eating of unhealthy foods, without the right nutrients, the body cannot properly protect, detoxify or restore itself

3. **Vaccines Increased** – they've doubled in number since 1991, which increased the load of toxic mercury, increased the frequency, and increased the probability of children receiving multiple vaccines in a single injection

4. **Ability to Detoxify Dwindled** – toxins that entered children's bodies over the past 15 to 20 years became more likely to stay there, due particularly to damage among millions of children to two important detoxification processes known as methylation and sulfation, which are responsible for removing mercury and other toxins.

Bock concludes that "These four catastrophic changes created a veritable perfect storm of physical and neurological insult, which struck hardest at our society's most vulnerable members: our children."[lxxv]

In Part I we have already mentioned quite a bit about the first couple of points made by Dr. Bock. While he does not claim that vaccines *cause* ADD/ADHD or other childhood diseases; he is stating that they add to the toxic load that our children are having a hard time removing from their bodies. And to point four, ability to detoxify, I have only begun to scratch the surface of the significance of this one (and have personally been affected by it).

Many genetic variations (called single nucleotide polymorphisms, SNPs, or "snips") exist in our bodies, most of which have existed for hundreds of years. But unfortunately the way that we have modified our food supply is making these variations "express" (become symptomatic) in some people where they never may have been significant, or they begin earlier in life, so that "diseases of aging" are now becoming diseases of younger people (arthritis, cardiovascular disease, diabetes, fibromyalgia, etc.).

A clear example of this is the 1992 mandatory folic acid fortification of the food supply in the United States (almost all processed flours and grains including processed foods *using* flours and grains, drinks, etc.). This fortification was done for one reason: to decrease neural tube defects in pregnancy due to folate deficiency. But clearly no one took genetics into consideration before making this decision.

Folate (in the form of Dihyrdofolate) is a naturally occurring vitamin in green leafy plants and other plant-foods. Folic acid is a synthetic derivative of folate and is broken down in a completely different way in our bodies (it takes a lot more work).

> Over 40% of the population has a genetic SNP variation, MTHFR, which slows down or prohibits our ability to break down folic acid. If folic acid can't be broken down (or is broken down super slowly), but keeps coming in with every bite of food, it builds up in our bodies. It can bind to and block folate receptors in our body and brain (so even if we eat the good and natural form of folate, it can't be used by our bodies). This can cause other problems with methylation, including causing an increase in homocysteine, as well as disrupting our ability to detoxify (our normal daily ability to get toxins from air, water, food and our environment *out* of our body).

If we only **ate** our folate-rich food, this artificial supplementation would not have ever been necessary! Green leafy vegetables (and other plant foods) provide folate, the naturally occurring substance, which our bodies can use much more readily and easily and which does not gum up these pathways. And while it has not been definitively proven, researchers are suspicious that this one substance, folic acid fortification of foods, can (together with increasing loads of immunizations and other childhood exposures) be contributive to the escalation of autism which began sharply in 1993 (remember, folic acid fortification began in 1992).

Is there also a genetic mutation associated with ADD susceptibility (as with folate pathways discussed above)? It is highly likely, but it is **not** an excuse or predestination. Repeatedly research has shown that just because you have a gene does not mean that the gene will express itself.

How we eat, move, supplement, and our environmental toxic exposures (stress, chemicals, etc.) are MORE important than our genes themselves!

So how a mother eats during pregnancy and how children eat and move throughout their lifetime play a role not just in whether ADD might express itself, but also how people with ADD can help their body naturally prevent the occurrence of the symptoms associated with it.

In all forms of ADD, healing is possible, but as the parent, you will need to stay on top of a child's nutrition and any exposure to toxic stimuli (environmental toxins). Medication is not necessarily the first or even best intervention to try for all children, even though many parents are pushed there by frustrated teachers. There is more information found in the last section: So Now What the Heck Do I Do?

There are many more ways that a person with ADD can be naturally treated and how those who interact with ADD can help (parents, teachers, etc.). To learn more about this condition, the research that is ongoing, and natural treatment options, please read resources available from Drs. Kenneth Bock, Natasha Campbell-McBride, and/or Daniel Amen.

[lxxi] Bock, Kenneth. Healing the New Childhood Epidemics: Autism, ADHD, Asthma, and Allergies: The Groundbreaking Program for the 4-A Disorders, Ballantine Books, 2008.
[lxxii] Amem. Daniel G. Healing ADD, The Berkley Publishing Group, 2013.
[lxxiii] Ibid.
[lxxiv] Campbell-McBride, Natasha. Gut And Psychology Syndrome - Natural Treatment for Autism, ADHD, Dyslexia, Dyspraxia, Depression and Schizophrenia, Medinform Publishing, 2012.
[lxxv] Bock, Kenneth Healing the New Childhood Epidemics: Autism, ADHD, Asthma, and Allergies: The Groundbreaking Program for the 4-A Disorders, Ballantine Books, 2008.

CHAPTER 16

OBESITY

What makes us fat?

Despite the continued call to "eat less and exercise more," this is not just a simple calories-in-calories-out model. Even Michelle Obama's *Let's Move* initiative stopped short of the whole story and only focused on fitness. The food industry would *love* to make it out to be purely a fitness issue. Remember, the food and beverages you consume contain messages that speak to your cells, hormones and brain. Junk food equals junk moods, obesity and disease.

Youth are increasingly becoming overweight and obese.

Among children and adolescents aged two through 19 years, 16.9% were obese and 31.8% were either overweight or obese.[lxxvi] The children aged two through five years had a 12.1% rate of obesity, children aged six through 11 years 18.0% rate, and adolescents 12 through 19 years an 18.4% rate. So, now that school aged children have higher rates of obesity and there are 22 studies that show that when weight goes up, the actual physical size and function of the brain goes down, we can conclude that increased weight is damaging our children's minds.

Obesity damages a child's ability to "do" school.

Obesity reduces physical activity and causes difficulty with routine tasks. It decreases the functioning in (damages) the prefrontal cortex. By doing so, it affects the ability to have forethought, judgment, impulse control, organization, planning, empathy and to learn from the mistakes you made.[lxxvii] Obese children may be at risk for both short-term health consequences[lxxviii] and long-term tracking of obesity to adulthood.[lxxix]

Obesity causes practical, everyday problems and leads to chronic diseases such as:

- Metabolic syndrome
- Type 2 diabetes
- Depression
- Alzheimer's disease
- Hypertension
- Heart disease, and
- Cancer

Food can be both the cause *and* the solution to the obesity epidemic.

When you use high quality, whole (unprocessed) foods, it is a solution. Dr. Mark Hyman summed it up: "Leave the food that man made; eat the food that God made." It's really that simple. When you use low quality processed and convenient foods, it contributes to obesity. The food we are eating today is not only higher in processed flour and sugar; it's altered through the hybridization of plants, the genetic modification of organisms (GMO), and is altered through the addition of chemicals and additives in amounts that we have never seen before.

Obesity is fostered by the toxic food environment found on most school campuses and unfortunately, in many family homes.

In North America, malnourished children are more likely to be overweight because they aren't getting enough of the right kinds of food to eat. So providing "free and reduced" school breakfasts and lunches may not solve (and in fact may be part of) the problem when those meals are truly not nutritious.

Malnutrition comes about from not getting sufficient nutrients from food consumed.

Just "grabbing a bite to eat" may not satisfy the needs of your body. Malnutrition that occurs at young ages makes a person more prone to obesity and chronic diseases.

Not all calories are created equally. If your lunch consists of a bag of Cheetos and a bottle of soda, it "fills" you up and shuts off your biological drive to seek calories (for a time), but you received little to nothing beneficial out of what you consumed.

Two pieces of white bread have about the same approximate caloric content of an apple. Can you think about what an apple might provide (think micronutrients) that the bread does not? Most micronutrients (vitamins, minerals, enzymes, antioxidants and phytonutrients) that exist in the bread are synthetic and were added back in *after* the plant was processed and turned into flour. Our bodies cannot readily use and absorb those synthetic nutrients as well as those that come straight from the whole plant. One such ingredient is folic acid, which will be discussed in several of these chapters as contributing to various diseases in some people.

All food and beverages consumed break down into a form of energy: a calorie. Thus, most of our school education has stopped here. But calories are information that speak to our brain, cells and hormones. Sugar, for instance, speaks directly to insulin. It tells it to store fat. When you consume more calories from macronutrients (protein, carbohydrates and fat) than your body needs, it stores them as fat. Yes, even excess protein becomes fat if your body doesn't need it. *This* is why many people get hung up on the eat less, exercise more model.

[lxxvi] Ogden CD, et al. "Prevalence and trends among overweight US children and adolescents." JAMA. 288(2002):1728-1732.

[lxxvii] Amen, Daniel G., Change Your Brain, Change Your Life, Three Rivers Press, 1998.

[lxxviii] Freedman DS et al. Cardiovascular risk factors and excess adiposity among overweight children and adolescents: the Bogalusa Heart Study. J Pediatr. 2007;150(1):12-17, e2

[lxxix] Singh AS et al. Tracking of childhood overweight into adulthood: a systematic review of the literature. Obes Rev. 2008;9(5):474-488.

CHAPTER 17

METABOLIC SYNDROME

Metabolic syndrome is the name for a group of risk factors that raise your risk for heart disease and other health problems, such as diabetes and stroke. It is present in 25 percent of Americans and has also been called syndrome X, insulin resistance syndrome or dysmetabolic syndrome. A diagnosis of metabolic syndrome is made if a person has any three of the following risk factors:[lxxx]

- A large waistline. This also is called abdominal obesity or "having an apple shape." Excess fat in the stomach area is a greater risk factor for heart disease than excess fat in other parts of the body, such as on the hips. [Waist circumference: at least 35 inches for women and at least 40 inches for men.]

- High fasting blood sugar (or you're on medicine to treat high blood sugar). Mildly high blood sugar may be an early sign of diabetes. [Fasting blood glucose at least 100 mg/dL]

- A high triglyceride level (or you're on medicine to treat high triglycerides). Triglycerides are a type of fat found in the blood. [Untreated serum triglycerides at least 150 mg/dL]

- High blood pressure (or you're on medicine to treat high blood pressure). Blood pressure is the force of blood pushing against the walls of your arteries as your heart pumps blood. If this pressure rises and stays high over time, it can damage your heart and lead to plaque buildup. [Blood pressure at least 135/85mmHg]

- A low HDL cholesterol level (or you're on medicine to treat low HDL cholesterol). HDL sometimes is called "good" cholesterol. This is because it helps remove cholesterol from your arteries. A low HDL cholesterol level raises your risk for heart disease. [HDL cholesterol lower than 40 mg/dL for men or 50 mg/dL for women.]

Kids are increasingly being diagnosed with metabolic syndrome. Their risk for heart disease, diabetes, and stroke increases with the number of metabolic risk factors they have. In general, a person who has metabolic syndrome is twice as likely to develop heart disease and five times as likely to develop diabetes as someone who doesn't have metabolic syndrome. **The risk of having metabolic syndrome is closely linked to overweight and obesity and a lack of physical activity.** Insulin resistance also may increase your risk for metabolic syndrome.[lxxxi]

Based on the National Institutes of Health's stated risks for metabolic syndrome, schools are contributing to the problem! School aged children are statistically becoming more overweight and obese (Section Three, Obesity). Food on school campuses contributes to weight gain and insulin resistance (Section One). Physical activity is diminishing on school campuses (Section Two, PE).

It is possible to prevent or delay metabolic syndrome, mainly with lifestyle changes. However, a healthy lifestyle is a lifelong commitment.[lxxxii]

Dr. Andrew Weil holds that the conventional medical recommendations for (or school diets that promote) a low-fat, high-carbohydrate diet to lower triglycerides and bring down cholesterol are dead wrong. He states, "Eating a diet high in the wrong kinds of carbohydrate and fat may actually elevate triglycerides and cholesterol."[lxxxiii] Instead, he recommends following an anti-inflammatory diet (and I strongly concur). The purpose of an anti-

98

inflammatory diet (or "way of eating") is to maintain a steady blood sugar (reducing glucose and insulin fluctuations) and reducing gut irritation and hormone reactions from food. You *could* eat this way for the rest of your life. It is not just a fad or a temporary fix. The following are general suggestions for following this way of eating:

- Eat smaller, more frequent meals to keep blood sugar from spiking (and therefore from insulin having to respond).

- Keep refined starches and sugars to a minimum, try to combine them in a meal with an overall low glycemic load* (also for the purpose of keeping a stable blood sugar). *More on glycemic load at the end of the book.

- Try to eat fats from whole plant food sources (e.g. nuts, seeds, avocado), minimize saturated fats (meat, dairy, coconut oil), reduce the use of oils (e.g. olive oil, walnut oil) and remove trans-fats (artificially created fats) (See Section One, Fat-Oils for more).

- Eat flax seeds and/or take Omega 3, EPA/DHA or krill oil supplements.

- Eat generous amounts of non-starchy vegetables, like broccoli, cauliflower, dark leafy greens, tomatoes, cucumbers, bell peppers, zucchini, asparagus, cabbage, Brussel sprouts, beans, radishes and spinach. More at: http://en.wikipedia.org/wiki/List_of_non-starchy_vegetables

- Eat foods high in magnesium, which has been shown to lower the incidence of metabolic syndrome,[lxxxiv] like whole grains, leafy green vegetables, as well as almonds, cashews and other nuts, avocados, lentils, beans, and soybeans.

[lxxx] Jankovic D, et al. "Prevalence of Endocrine Disorders in Morbidly Obese Patients and the Effects of Bariatric Surgery on Endocrine and Metabolic Parameters." *Obesity Surgery* 22(1)(2011): 62-69.
[lxxxi] What is Metabolic Syndrome? National Heart, Lung and Blood Institute, http://www.nhlbi.nih.gov/health/health-topics/topics/ms/; available July 30, 2014.
[lxxxii] Ibid.
[lxxxiii] Andrew Weil, MD. *Metabolic Syndrome.*

http://www.drweil.com/drw/u/ART03193/Metabolic-Syndrome.html; accessed July 30, 2014.

[lxxxiv] He K et al. "Magnesium intake and the metabolic syndrome: epidemiologic evidence to date." J Cardiometab Syndr. 2006 Fall;1(5):351-5.

CHAPTER 18

TYPE 2 DIABETES

Diabetes occurs hand-in-hand with obesity. It is possible for skinny people to have diabetes, but these are generally people who are "skinny fat" (they are thin, but their fat level is still over healthy levels). We experienced the start of a diabetes epidemic between 1990 and 1998 when we had a 33% increase in rates.[lxxxv] As many as 11% of American adults are now diabetic,[lxxxvi] with over 150,000 young people diagnosed. An astonishing one in three born in the year 2000 is at risk of developing Type 2 diabetes (and one in two African Americans, Native Americans and Hispanic Americans) in his or her lifetime, unless there are significant changes made to diet and activity levels.

Type 1 diabetes used to be referred to as *juvenile onset* or *insulin-dependent* as it develops in children and renders them unable to produce sufficient insulin. It compromises approximately 5% of diagnosed cases of diabetes.

As many as one-third of American adults have prediabetes, which used to be called impaired glucose tolerance, impaired fasting glucose or borderline diabetes. The majority of people with prediabetes are generally without symptoms. Long term damage may already be occurring in the body, especially to the heart and circulatory system in prediabetics. Weight loss can prevent or delay this onset.

Type 2 diabetes used to be referred to as *adult onset*, and as opposed to Type 1 diabetes, occurred in adults, ages 40 and up. That is now not the case as 45% of newly diagnosed Type 2 diabetes cases are in children. It is the most common form of diabetes (with approximately 95% of diagnosed cases). Type 2 diabetics have lost control of blood glucose levels, leading to insulin resistance—and all of this stems from dietary habits.

For children, obesity and resultant diabetes are not necessarily a choice.

Food provided in school cafeterias and fast food put on the table in the name of dinner not only contribute to their present status, but to the dietary habits they are likely to follow for a lifetime.

Common complications of diabetes:

- 2-to-4 times risk of death from heart disease
- 2-to-4 times risk of stroke
- More than 70% of people with diabetes have high blood pressure
- Leading cause of blindness in adults
- Leading cause of end-stage kidney disease
- 60-70% of diabetics suffer mild to severe nervous system damage

Modern drugs and surgery really offer no cure. At best, current drugs help to maintain a reasonably functional lifestyle, but these drugs will never offer substantial improvement. As a consequence, diabetics face a lifetime of drugs and medications, making diabetes an enormously costly disease. The economic toll of diabetes [in the U.S.] is over 130 billion dollars a year.[lxxxvii]

Isn't Diabetes Genetic?

Many children are born with genes that make it possible for them to develop Type 1 diabetes, but many of them never do. Even among identical twins, when one twin has Type 1 diabetes, the other has less than a 40 percent chance of having it.[lxxxviii] Apparently the difference is found in their environment, particularly in the foods the child is exposed to early in life, viral infections, and most likely other factors. Genes play a similar role in Type 2 diabetes. If kids eat the same foods as their parents do or did, they are very likely going to develop a similar disease as their parents. There is much evidence to show that changing diet and lifestyle can significantly cut the odds that diabetes will occur.

The first nutrient to eliminate in an effort to avoid diabetes is processed carbohydrates.

Carbohydrates are a very large category of plant-based foods that are macronutrients and provide energy to our body. But getting energy would be a good thing, right? Let's just say that some carbohydrates create "clean burning energy" and others just provide sludge.

Clean-burning energy is provided by whole, unrefined and unaltered carbohydrates. In fact, they should be the staple of our diet: fruit, vegetables, unprocessed non-gluten-containing grains (preferably the ancient grains e.g. rice, quinoa, kamut, amaranth, faro, teff) and beans.

Sludge energy is made from a plant that has been processed, stripped of all micronutrients, fluffed up (by adding a few synthetic nutrients back in), dressed up and packaged in a pretty box, bag or container. In fact, we might call this sludge "anti-energy" because it leeches energy in your body by creating inflammation. Most flours, sugars, cereals, pastas and other foods found in the middle of a grocery store fall into this category. Now there are some flours, cereals and pastas that are made from quality ingredients (e.g. non-gluten-containing flours and not a lot of "extras") and can be eaten on occasion without causing inflammation in your body.

The Making of Diabetes in Our Bodies:

All carbohydrates break down into glucose to create energy, as mentioned above. But sugar and processed carbohydrates have a higher glycemic index, that is, they cause the blood glucose to rise faster, which in turn causes insulin to rise (because it's insulin's job to move glucose out of the bloodstream and into our cells).

When insulin levels are elevated, we store and cannot release fat. So if you are (or your child is) eating a diet high in processed carbohydrates all day long, you are simply storing and never releasing or burning previously stored fat. And burning out your insulin receptors while you're at it—they get tired of having to work all day, day-in-and-day-out; don't you?

Healing Our Bodies Before and After a Diabetes Diagnosis

Learning how to correct the *cause* and not just treat the symptom (e.g. insulin sensitivity) is what is necessary. Neal Barnard, M.D. has successfully shown that he is able to prevent and reverse diabetes using diet – changing how people eat to prevent and reverse what has previously been called a chronic and irreversible disease. And this is *nothing* like the diet promoted by the American Diabetes Association (ADA) and lackluster results found from it.[lxxxix]

To learn how to prevent and/or reverse Type 2 diabetes in yourself or a family member, I encourage you to read Dr. Neal Barnard's *Program for Reversing Diabetes*, published in 2007 by Rodale Books. You will not be disappointed and you will *not* be hungry!

[lxxxv] Mokdad AH et al. "Diabetes trends in the US 1990-1998." Diabetes Care 23(2000):1278-1783.

[lxxxvi] Centers for Disease Control and Prevention (2011). Numbers of Americans with Diabetes Rises to Nearly 26 Million; http://www.cdc.gov/media/releases/2011/p0126_diabetes.html; available July 26, 2014.

[lxxxvii] Centers for Disease Control and Prevention. "National diabetes fact sheet:

general information and national estimates on diabetes in the United States, 2000." Atlanta, GA: Centers for Disease Control and Prevention, 2000.

[lxxxviii] Knipp M et al. "Environmental Triggers and Determinants of Type 1 Diabetes," *Diabetes* 54, suppl 2 (December 2005):S125-36.

[lxxxix] Barnard RJ et al. "Diet and Exercise in the Treatment of NIDDM: The Need for Early Emphasis," *Diabetes Care* 17(1994):1469-72.

CHAPTER 19

DEPRESSION AND DEMENTIA

Depression is one of the greatest killers of our time.

It is a disorder of the brain and it affects 50 million Americans at some point. There are a variety of causes, including genetic, environmental, psychological, and biochemical factors. Symptoms can include:

- Sadness
- Loss of interest or pleasure in activities you used to enjoy
- Change in weight
- Difficulty sleeping or oversleeping
- Energy loss
- Feelings of worthlessness, and/or
- Thoughts of death or suicide.

If your child is suffering from depression, he or she is "normal," but does need help. Don't start with drugs (they have actually been shown to be no more effective than a placebo[xc]), but start by getting his or her diet right. Gluten can literally make people who are sensitive have psychotic episodes (not kidding!). Try removing gluten and dairy because it's been proven that their removal can make an extreme change in cognitive health.

Depression is not something to ignore. It is a risk factor for:

- Alzheimer's disease
- Heart disease
- Cancer
- Obesity and
- Diabetes.

Sugar imbalances can mimic a form of depression. When in the "low" of an imbalance, a child (or adult) can become very agitated, irritable or quiet and sullen, with little energy. Many of our kids go through their whole day this way: up and down, up and down from one sugar high to the next. Let's give their brain chemistry a chance of success and provide consistent, solid and nutritious food so that the hormones that control the brain get the right message.

Genes can also play a role in depression but do not have to. We have the ability to turn our genes on and off (food and lifestyle can do that). First, work to improve your child's diet, and seek testing from his or her pediatrician or a functional medicine practitioner that might be able to help you rule out an organic cause. Oftentimes the neurotransmitters (the "feel good" hormones) are out of balance and just need some help (which can be done nutritionally and with supplements).

In Chapter 15, I introduced the concept of *folic acid fortification* of our food supply and how it is creating problems for a large portion of the population. Here is how it can relate to depression:

- MTHFR is a genetic variation, one that between 40-50% of the population has. It can decrease our ability to process folic acid, among other things.

- Folic acid fortification can cause a buildup of folic acid (a synthetic version of folate) in the body. This folic acid then blocks folate receptor sites and *causes* a folate deficiency.

- Folate deficiencies can further cause Tetrahydrobiopterin (BH4) deficiencies (folate is needed for the creation of BH4 in the body).

- BH4, in turn, is a cofactor essential for the production of neurotransmitters (the "feel good" and sleep hormones): serotonin, melatonin, dopamine, norepinephrine and epinephrine.

- Decreased BH4 = Decreased neurotransmitter production.

Symptoms of neurotransmitter deficiency can include:

- Sleep difficulties: problems falling asleep, waking frequently in the middle of the night, can't fall asleep after waking at night.

- Craving and overconsumption of refined carbohydrates (creating a vicious cycle!).

- Hard time dealing with life changes.

- Difficulty relaxing, tension.

- Fatigue even during the morning.

- Lack of concentration.

- Difficulty losing weight.

- Eating too much sugar.

- Depression.

- Feeling taken advantage of by others.

In turn, dementia is the loss of mental functions, such as thinking, memory, and reasoning and is severe enough to interfere with a person's daily functioning.

Dementia is not a disease itself, but rather a group of symptoms that are caused by various diseases or conditions. Symptoms can also include changes in personality, mood, and behavior. In some cases, the dementia can be treated and cured because the cause is treatable. Examples of this include dementia caused by substance abuse (illicit drugs and alcohol), combinations of prescription medications, and *hormone or vitamin imbalances.*

In some cases, although the person may appear to have dementia, a severe depression can be causing the symptoms. This is known as pseudo-dementia (false dementia) and is highly treatable. In most cases, however, true dementia cannot be cured.

Dementia develops when the parts of the brain that are involved with learning, memory, decision-making, and language are affected by one or more of a variety of infections or diseases. The most common cause of dementia is Alzheimer's disease, but there are as many as 50 other known causes. Most of these causes, however, are very rare.

Alzheimer's disease is expected to triple in the next 25 years.

There is no cure on the horizon. *The disease starts at least 30 years before any symptoms are recognized.* The reality is that *there is no time to wait*. It affects 50% of adults over the age of 85. The **best prevention** is to decrease illnesses that increase risk, such as obesity, heart disease, depression and sleep apnea. If you don't exercise at least twice per week, you have an increased risk. Untreated depression doubles the risk in women and more than quadruples it in men. The biggest take home: don't wait to take care of your health.

So, in summary, depression can be caused by many things, but biochemical factors are among them, which includes food, exposure to artificial food coloring and additives, a lack of necessary vitamins and minerals for healthy brain function, and more.

Depression, dementia and even Alzheimer's can be caused by, and therefore prevented by, food!

So, let's work to correct that and give our kids a fighting chance.

[xc] Emslie GJ et al. A Double-blind, Randomized, Placebo-Controlled Trial of Fluoxetine in Children and Adolescents With Depression. Arch Gen Psychiatry. 1997;54(11):1031-1037.

CHAPTER 20

HYPERTENSION AND HEART DISEASE

Hypertension is a condition of chronic high blood pressure. Normal blood pressure is between 100/60 and 140/90 mmHg. High blood pressure is said to be present if it is often at or above 140/90 mmHg.

Blood pressure is driven by two physical forces — the one from the heart as it pumps blood into the arteries and through the circulatory system, and the other from the arteries as they resist this blood flow. Blood pressure changes from minute to minute and is affected by activity and rest, body temperature, diet, emotional state, posture, and medications.

While hypertension is far more common among adults, the rate among kids is on the rise, a trend that experts link to the increase in childhood obesity. Many kids and teens with high blood pressure have no other health problems but do have a family history of hypertension and an unhealthy lifestyle — a bad diet, excess weight, stress, and insufficient physical activity.

Hypertension is classified as either primary (essential) hypertension or secondary hypertension; about 90–95% of cases are categorized as primary hypertension, which means high blood pressure with no obvious underlying medical cause.[xci] The remaining 5–10% of cases (secondary hypertension) are caused by other conditions that affect the kidneys, arteries, heart or endocrine system.

Having high blood pressure puts someone at a higher risk for stroke, heart attack, kidney failure, loss of vision, and atherosclerosis (hardening of the arteries). A moderately high arterial blood pressure is associated with a shortened life expectancy while mild elevation is not. Dietary and lifestyle changes can improve blood pressure control and decrease the risk of health complications.

There are conflicting research studies and conflicting beliefs about *what exactly causes heart disease*, but there is agreement that it is food and a lack of physical activity. One camp says it's saturated fat, yet another says it is high blood glucose (sugar or simple carbohydrates like bread) in the presence of fat (think jelly donut). But while they are arguing over what might be the exact cause, there are pioneers like Dr. Dean Ornish, who are using food to heal people from heart disease. So once again, as in many chronic diseases, **food is the cause *and* the cure**!

Important risk factors for heart disease that you can do something about are:

- High blood pressure
- High blood cholesterol
- Diabetes
- Smoking
- Being overweight, and
- Being physically inactive.[xcii]

Being overweight in adolescence increases the rates of future heart disease. A prospective study looked at the effect of overweight adolescents on future rates of coronary heart disease (CHD). And there is a projected increase in the prevalence of obese 35-year-olds in 2020 to a range of 30-37% in men and 34-44% in women. As a consequence of this increase in obesity, an increase in the incidence of heart disease and in the total

112

number of heart disease events and deaths is projected to occur in young adulthood.[xciii]

I previously discussed how the fortification of *folic acid* in our food supply is creating problems for a large portion of the population in the areas of detoxification (the ability to remove chemicals and toxins from our body) and methylation. Methylation is a series of very important biochemical reactions in the body that are responsible for overall good health. A properly functioning methylation pathway has life rewarding health benefits including:

- proper brain function

- healthy detoxification

- DNA protection

- a healthy, normal, non-premature aging process.

In a large portion of the population, folic acid blocks folate receptors and *creates* a folate deficiency.
Because folic acid can gum up and block folate receptors, it decreases our ability to absorb and use folate (the natural vitamin from green leafy vegetables and other plant-based foods), creating a folate deficiency, which was the very reason the government made folic acid fortification mandatory in the beginning (a circular way of saying, that while it worked in a certain portion of the population, it is creating much worse problems in a very large part of the population, including many of our children).

Folate deficiencies can cause:

- Neural-tube and other mid-line defects

- Methylation pathway problems, which can lead to problems with brain function, normal DNA replication and premature aging.

113

- Tetrahydrobiopterin (BH4) deficiencies, which may lead to MANY other medical problems because BH4 is a very important cofactor in many biochemical reactions.

- Buildup (or increase) of homocysteine.

Homocysteine is an amino acid in the blood. The American Heart Association states that too much homocysteine is related to a higher risk of coronary heart disease, stroke and peripheral vascular disease (fatty deposits in peripheral arteries).

As many as 40% of the population of children (those who have the MTHFR genetic variation) are being fed in a way that puts them at greater risk of developing a risk for coronary artery disease, stroke and/or peripheral vascular disease.

Heart disease is as it sounds: a disease of your heart. Symptoms can range from rising and falling blood pressure, chest pain, dizziness, shortness of breath, fatigue, stress, worry and depression, persistent coughing or wheezing, swelling of the ankles and feet, and can lead to stroke, heart attack and even death.

The American Heart Association reported that 12.8% of men and 10.1% of women ages 20-39 currently have heart disease and reported that, of cardiovascular risk factors in 12-19 year olds, 91.5% have a "Poor" rating on the *Healthy Diet Score* (rating of food consumed, based on criteria for ideal cardiovascular health) and only 36.5% have an "Ideal" rating for physical activity (8.2% "Poor" and 55.3% "Intermediate").[xciv]

So, if our diets suck so badly, where did we all learn to eat this way?

Hmm … our own school education (much of the health curricula is underwritten by food industry), mass marketing of convenient and fast food (think of the commercials that come on during kids' television programming), and a lack of quality in the food that we are getting today (as much of it has been altered through hybridization, genetic modification, pesticide and chemical spraying and more) just may be the sources and cause.

How do we *change?*

Often the *how* has to be proceeded by a *why* in order to make sustainable change. Have you read enough about kids being put at risk (either immediately or in the long run) for ADD/ADHD, obesity, metabolic syndrome, Type 2 diabetes, depression, dementia, hypertension, and heart disease to want to make a change? I hope so. I sure did. It's what has been pushing me to write this book and what will continue to push me to talk to moms and dads just like you across the country.

Dr. Ornish has created a scientifically proven system to prevent and even reverse heart disease without drugs or surgery. The same program would substantially reduce the risk of developing any of the other mentioned chronic diseases and even help prevent many cancers. The only difference between the prevention and the reversal plans is the amount of cholesterol allowed because someone who already has heart disease needs to work hard to break down the buildup already accumulated. We make cholesterol in our bodies, so we do not need to ingest cholesterol as its own food group. However, we do need (especially young people absolutely need) healthy fat in our diet (addressed in Section One), but coming from whole plants, including nuts and seeds is much healthier than oils and processed fats.

If there is a scientifically proven method of preventing chronic disease, why don't our schools teach our children how to eat and live this way *and provide food to the same end*?

A pretty good question that many of us need to start asking a lot more. To learn more for your family, you can read Dr. Dean Ornish's *Program for Reversing Heart Disease.*

[xci] Carretero OA, Oparil S (January 2000). "Essential hypertension. Part I: definition and etiology". Circulation 101 (3): 329–35

[xcii] What Are the Risk Factors for Heart Disease? NIH, National Heart, Lung and Blood Institute; http://www.nhlbi.nih.gov/health/educational/hearttruth/lower-risk/risk-factors.htm; available August 7, 2014.

[xciii] Bibbins-Domingo K et al. *Adolescent Overweight and Future Adult Coronary Heart Disease*, N Engl J Med 2007;357:2371-9.

[xciv] Go AS, Mozaffarian D et al. Heart disease and stroke statistics—2014 update. http://circ.ahajournals.org/content/129/3/e28; available August 6, 2014.

CHAPTER 21

TYPES OF CANCER

Cancer has been viewed as the bogeyman that we are "doomed" to get if we have a certain gene (or family history). There is much fear; but that fear can be replaced with hope when we have reliable knowledge. T. Colin Campbell, PhD said that,

"Lack of knowledge encourages fear, an emotion that seems to permeate every level of what has now become a cancer industry."

Cancer is not some out-of-this-world invader. It exists in all of our bodies at all times. The problem is when our immune system gets so compromised that the cancers are allowed to grow (multiply) and spread.

Cancer is a process typically considered and studied as a sequence of three stages: initiation (Stage 1), promotion (Stage 2) and progression (Stage 3). Initiation begins the process, promotion pushes it along, and progression describes the more serious stage of cancer, as it begins to spread from its primary site into other tissue sites.

It has always been a concern that cancer was caused by chemicals found in our food, water and environment.

As a result, there was considerable pressure to identify which of the 80,000-100,000 environmental synthetic chemicals might cause cancer. Government-led research programs tested chemicals and regulations were put into place. In 1958, an amendment was added to the food and drug regulations, called the Delaney Amendment. Under the Delaney Amendment, "… no additive was deemed safe if it is found [in 'appropriate' tests] to induce cancer when ingested by man or animal …" The Amendment required zero tolerance; no amount of carcinogen could be added to food. Now that's what I'm talking about! "First, do no harm!"

But, of the 80,000-100,000 environmental chemicals already out there, which are carcinogenic? It has been impossible to test them all. It would be near impossible to eliminate them all. The focus on the chemicals has diverted attention from other critical causes like nutrient imbalances. The experimental requirements are seriously flawed: testing in humans not allowed (lab animal extrapolation not always accurate).

Zero tolerance was no longer considered reasonable, so in 1996 the Delaney Amendment was repealed. The current tolerance level is one in one million cancer cases allowed. The focus on single chemicals as primary causes of cancer remains with us.

The Causes of Cancer

- Any factor or condition that favors cancer development at any of its stages.
- Chemicals have been shown to initiate or promote cancer (Stage 1-2).
- Viruses have been shown to initiate or promote cancer (Stage 1-2).
- Family history (genetics); inheritance of mutated genes.
- Excessive sunlight/radiation may initiate or promote cancer (Stage 1-2).

- Stress (compromises in some way the very complex immune system that otherwise keeps the development of cancer under control)—may act during any of the stages.

Historically, chemical carcinogens and genes were blamed for cancer initiation (Stage 1). But the reality is, the body has many mechanisms for trying to break down those chemicals and excreting them (through feces and urine). And as previously stated in the chapter on diabetes, genes may predispose, but they do not determine whether or not you will have a disease: *your diet, lifestyle and exposures contribute significantly.*

Promotion (Stage 2) may be a year(s) long process. But thankfully, this stage of cancer development has been shown to be reversible under certain conditions.

Nutritional Influences

- Low dietary animal protein (less than 10% of daily caloric intake) decreases both Initiation (Stage 1) and Promotion (Stage 2) of cancer, but its effect on Promotion (Stage 2) are most pronounced.

- Nutrition activity during Promotion (Stage 2) strongly indicates that cancer development can be controlled, perhaps even reversed, by nutritional means. Studies show the ability to turn cancer on and off, even at relatively advanced stages of the disease by the manipulation of protein intake.

Other Nutritional Effects and Experimental Cancer

- Protein intake that's greater than 10% of daily caloric intake acts swiftly to affect carcinogen metabolism (tumor growth).

- Plant based proteins do not increase pre-cancer development, even at 20% of dietary calories.

- High fat increased early pancreatic cancer.

- Low carotenoids increased early liver cancer.

- High fat increased transplanted mammary tumors.

Cancer Prevention through Food:

- Less fat (see Section One—the chapter on oils and fats)

- Less animal protein

- More plant protein

- More carotenoids—most commonly found in orange colored fruits and vegetables (e.g. sweet potatoes, carrots, carrot and tomato juice, pumpkin, cantaloupe and apricots); also found in spinach and broccoli

The biggest problem with human cancer studies is that nutritional effects are misrepresented. In observational studies, statistical adjustments are used for confounding effects. In randomized clinical trials (the "gold standard" of research), they are only directly testing the independent effects of *one* agent and we know that foods and nutrients act synergistically in our bodies (e.g. eating an apple for vitamin c is so much more effective than taking a vitamin c pill because there are other nutrients in the apple that help the nutrient being studied be more effective).

Also, in large studies of breast cancer, the relationship to animal foods, not just total fat, is critical. In the *Nurse's Health Study*[xcv] they reported that the altering of the level of dietary fat had "no influence" on breast cancer development. But in fact, a decrease in dietary fat was accompanied by a *higher* protein consumption (primarily lean animal protein), which would otherwise offset benefits of decreased fat diets. In this study, fruit and vegetable consumption remained unchanged, and low, for all groups.

Breast Cancer Risk Factors Keyed to Diet[xcvi]

As each of these factors *increases,* breast cancer risks either ↑or ↓:

- Age at menarche (start of menstrual cycle) (later start, breast cancer risk ↓)

- Body weight (higher the weight, breast cancer risk ↑)

- Consumption of meat (higher consumption, breast cancer risk ↑), grain (higher consumption, breast cancer risk ↓) and legumes (higher consumption, breast cancer risk ↓)

Plant foods tend to decrease, while animal foods tend to increase breast cancer risks. It is the *full complement* of nutrients in foods that plays a role in breast (and most likely other) cancer development.

Main lesson learned from the examples of dietary fat and breast cancer:

1. Total fat, alone, has no effect on breast cancer risk.

2. Neither is there evidence that animal protein, alone, effects breast cancer risk.

3. BEST HYPOTHESIS: Decreased consumption of animal-based foods and/or increased consumption of whole, unprocessed plant-based foods (as opposed to supplements of individual nutrients or processed plant foods) decreases breast cancer risk.

If you would like additional resources to help you learn how to use food to fight cancer, I highly recommend Neal Barnard M.D. and Jennifer Reilly RD's book *The Cancer Survivor's Guide* (2008, Healthy Living Publications). It does a really good job of helping you understand what to eat, and includes recipes and support.

PART IV

SO NOW WHAT THE HECK DO I DO?

First of all, please take a deep breath. I know how overwhelming and painful some of this can feel: lies, deceit, false advertising, profit-at-tolerable-risk, guilt …yes, yes, and yes! It can get to the point where you don't know who or what to trust, what to eat, or what's safe to feed your kids. I've been there! And I want to help you choose as wisely as possible, provide additional tools to assist you, and help you feel confident that it is possible to feed your family nutritious food, on a budget, that also tastes good.

But change can take time—developing new habits, breaking food addictions and finding new foods that you enjoy. We are so used to *convenience* and health isn't always convenient. But I want to teach you short cuts and ways to bulk-prepare so you always have things you can grab.

It is possible that you and/or your children may be addicted to sugar or may even have a bacterial or yeast overgrowth in your intestines that screams for sugar! You may have blood sugar imbalances that cause spikes and crashes, which cause you to crave more sugar. There are over 6,000 food substances in America and over 80% of them have sugar added. Sugar (as well as cheese, meat and other products) are addicting! They either have in them, or create in your brain, morphine-like substances that keep you coming back for more. So give your new habits time, patience and persistence. Your long term health will be the payoff.

The best things that you can do for your family is to be willing to step out, try something new and make it a family priority—get the kids involved. Yes, it takes more time to involve the kids, but oh! What an amazing, hands-on approach to getting them interested, involved and *helping*!

122

By getting your children in the kitchen, you can teach them about the things you are learning and how they too can be a part of making food that will truly nourish our bodies and brains! And by involving your kids now, as they mature and make more of their food choices, it's more likely they will be to make the best choices possible *and* they may even positively influence their peers (ripple effect!). Lastly, you might have little activists who want to become involved in school and or government policy change.

Please use any/all of the resources in this chapter. You will be able to find additional resources at http://AngelaGriffithsDC.com/HealtheChildren. And please, if you think of additional information or skills that would better assist you in this process, do leave a comment through the website. It is from your feedback that I will be able to continue to generate more resources that might assist you and many more moms, dads and grandparents just like you!

[xcv] Willett et al. *J Am Med Assoc* 1992
[xcvi] World Cancer Research Fund Reports, 1997

CHAPTER 22

STARTING AT HOME

The health of our children, and of our country, is at risk. We have been fed misinformation from the food industry as well as our government (as their track record shows them to stand behind big business rather than the health of its citizenry). The diets that we have all been encouraged to eat by the USDA, American Diabetes Association, American Heart Association and more have all promoted inflammation—the very inflammation that is at the root of the diseases that they stand to "prevent."

No one is looking after the *health* of your family except you!

"Health care" has become about acute and emergency care as well as disease management. Prescription medications aren't curing diseases or even decreasing the inflammation; they are just delaying death, covering up one symptom and replacing it with two or three more. We've "accepted" a lesser quality of living in exchange for more years.

Remember, our health starts with our food. As Hippocrates said, *"Let food be thy medicine and let medicine be thy food."* Ancient physicians understood how to heal. Current physicians have accepted the application of pharmaceuticals to mask symptoms. They are not even taught about nutrition in medical school. Where did we go wrong?

Food caused it and food can stop it! The answers are glaringly simple but their implementation is less so, but only because we have become so accustomed to convenience, fast food and even faster fixes (e.g. take a pill and "make it go away!"). Most chronic diseases (obesity, metabolic syndrome, Type 2 diabetes, hypertension, heart disease) started and are fueled by inflammation. An anti-inflammatory diet can turn them around. Steps for implementing an anti-inflammatory diet for your family can be found in the following pages.

Diseases are not "just a matter of genetics." It is possible to have a gene for a chronic disease, but that gene only "expresses" itself when your diet, lifestyle and toxic exposures allow it to manifest. Studies have shown immigrants adapt to the diseases of their new country rather than those of the country of their birth and genetic ancestry. So logic dictates it is more about how they change their diets when immigrating to a new country rather than their genes. Genes change over thousands of years, not one generation.

In modern times this can also be seen by the "exportation" of the *Standard American Diet (SAD)*. When one country's lifestyle and food habits are adopted by another country (e.g. McDonald's, Kentucky Fried Chicken and other fast food chains moving into China), the chronic diseases common in America begin to increase in those countries as well.

Do you want to find true health? When children are fed clean diets from birth, they have higher levels of immunity and less risk for chronic disease. Once chronic disease manifests, it is possible to lessen medication and even reverse symptoms of disease through clean living. However, you must understand that once you have a chronic disease, while you may eat to reverse symptoms and improve health indicators, you are always at risk of that disease returning *if you return to your previous ways of eating*.

125

True health is achieved by a series of good choices made repeatedly over time, not by a temporary period of healthy eating. However, every meal is a chance to make a healthier choice, so don't be discouraged if you make one bad choice. Drink some water and start over again.

Health through clean living is possible for everyone. But you may need to partner with a functional medicine practitioner or health coach to find out if you have present levels of inflammation, to learn new habits and how to crowd out harmful food choices. Many people respond to food and lifestyle changes alone. If you find that your body is "stubborn" (as mine was) either due to chronic dieting, nutrient deficiencies, hormone imbalances, food sensitivities, etc., you may need to work with a functional medicine practitioner to diagnose and correct these issues.

All food is hormonal messages sent directly to our cells. All calories are *not* created equal! And the calories that we consume are not just "energy"; they actually talk to our cells, to our hormones, and to our fat! That's right—our food sends messages throughout our body. Do you think that an apple with some almond butter and a piece of fried chicken say the same thing (even though they might contain the same amount of calories)? No way! The apple and nut butter set our body up for success, the fried chicken … well, not so much.

Good, Better to Best—it's like gradually climbing a ladder. If you are new to clean living, strive to do *better* than you did last month or last year. The more you strive for clean living, the better you optimize your health. Take it step by step.

If the whole idea of learning to eat more plants than animal foods is new to you, if you grew up on a fast food diet yourself and are feeling slightly overwhelmed at the prospect of change, start with the GOOD section that follows. Stay with that alone for a while (maybe even a few years) until you feel like you have the swing of things. Together, these suggestions will help you transition your family from the *Standard American Diet (SAD)* to an Anti-Inflammatory Diet that will promote better health for each of you.

If you have been introducing plant-based foods into your family's diet for a while and are ready to take the next step, read on through the BETTER section that follows. You might hang out there for a year or two.

If you feel like you're ready to take a leap and bring your whole family with you, keep reading on to the BEST section that follows. Remember, it's all a matter of degrees. If you bounce back to the GOOD section, you are still doing better than Frankenstein-like-food-substances. So, don't kick yourself for trying. Keep working at it.

GOOD – a matter of scale

Start with the list below but don't treat it as an "all or nothing." In other words, don't let it overwhelm you and don't feel that if you "can't do it all, you shouldn't do any." Start by learning how to cook at home more. Find some new, healthier recipes that appeal to you. Try to eat a few more vegetables every day and maybe add in one or two new ones a week.

If work or schedules dictate that you eat "out" a lot, learn how to make better choices and to order what you want rather than accepting how they present it on the menu. Make it fun! We are supposed to enjoy our food. Let's learn once again how to eat to nourish our bodies rather than to feed our emotions, shall we?

Clean Living, a Daily Choice

1. **Eat a wide variety of whole, natural foods.**
   Think about *eating from the rainbow* at every meal. Foods with natural color (blue, red, orange, green) offer more

antioxidants, phytonutrients and vitamins. Fruits and vegetables contain fiber that help you feel "full," and they keep your bowel movements regular, which gets waste out of your body and helps you stay healthy. You can find a sample of a phytonutrient rainbow on the resources page at: http://angelagriffithsdc.com/resources/.

2. **Choose water at every possible opportunity.** You might start carrying a bottle with you and send one to school with your child. Choose water over other liquids during meals (although it is better to consume your water between meals and not to drink heavy during a meal). A good goal is three to four liters (12-16 cups) of water per day, depending on your body size, sweat rate and amount of time spent exercising.

3. **Eat to stabilize blood sugar.** Eat more frequent meals to start, every 2-3 hours; combine a healthy fat, protein and carbohydrate with every meal (e.g. black beans, rice and avocado or guacamole).

4. **Choose whole grains** (e.g. quinoa, amaranth, millet) **or starchy vegetables** (e.g. sweet potato, butternut squash, etc.) **as starchy carbohydrate sources to replace processed foods.**

5. **Eat high quality food; it becomes you!** ("You are what you eat" -- literally!)

6. **Try to walk every day.** Walking as if walking the dog, as opposed to race-walking, helps to reset your primitive brain and can calm your adrenals, helping your body heal from daily stresses.

Supercharged!

I hope that by implementing these clean living principles you begin to feel more energy, think a little more clearly, and develop a new passion for your future. Clean, wholesome food has helped me to heal and survive. My deepest hope is that it can for you too! Give it some time though. It took you *how* many years to get to your present state of dis-ease? It can take some patience to work yourself back out of that.

BETTER – a matter of scale

If you are ready to take your clean living to the next level and continue to strive for healthy with and for your family members, hopefully you already read through and are familiar with the last section (GOOD), are putting those steps into play on a regular basis and are ready to move onto the next list.

Clean Living, a Daily Choice and Commitment

1. **Cook more meals at home.** This way you know the quality of the ingredients that you are using as well as what fats, oils or enhancers are added or avoided.

2. **Eat lots of fruits and vegetables, especially the bright colored ones** (eat from the "rainbow"). Fruits and vegetables contain fiber, antioxidants and phytonutrients that help promote health and prevent disease.

3. **Eat legumes** (peas, beans and lentils). Beans are high in antioxidants, fiber, protein, B vitamins, iron, magnesium, potassium, copper and zinc. Eating beans regularly may decrease the risk of diabetes, heart disease, colorectal cancer, and they help with weight management. Beans are hearty, helping you feel full so you will tend to eat less. (*Note*: if you have not regularly been consuming beans, start slowly, gradually eating them daily.) If your body has difficulty digesting beans at the start, begin slowly. You can also pre-soak beans if you are making your own (discard the rinse water), cook them with a three-inch piece of kombu (a type of seaweed) or really rinse a can of beans before you use it

129

(throw away the water it was canned in, pour into a strainer, and continue to rinse with fresh water).

4. **Avoid folic acid,** the synthetic version of methyl-folate, which can bind to and block folate receptor sites in your body. Folate is essential and deficiencies can be very serious. Instead, seek to get lots of natural folate (which converts easily to methyl-folate in your body) from green leafy vegetables and other plant-based foods. Always consult with a medical professional, qualified to advise you on nutrition, prior to adding supplements.

5. **Salt your food to a pleasant taste.** Himalayan or Celtic Sea salt is healthier than processed table salt; use fresh herbs to your heart's content.

6. **Avoid gluten.** Gluten can create inflammation in your stomach (and intestines), nerves, joints, muscles and even brain. It's not worth the risk. None of us *need* gluten, but many of us suffer as a result of consuming it. But remember, just because something is gluten-free, does *not* mean it is healthy. It can still contain other ingredients such as fillers, chemicals and/or oils that are inflammatory. Resources for learning how to become gluten-free can be found at www.AngelaGriffithsDC.com/HealtheChildren.

7. **Eat sugar minimally.** Remember, stabilizing the blood sugar is our goal; if you absolutely need to sweeten a little something now and then, Grade B maple syrup, raw coconut, coconut sugar or raw honey are healthier options (but still unhealthy in excess).

8. **Avoid High Fructose Corn Syrup (HFCS).** It has been shown to create many gastro-intestinal and other problems, even altering your body's metabolism by blocking methylation and sulfation pathways (leading to brain, memory, neurological, DNA repair and genetic problems). This happens when HFCS breaks down into ethanol in our bodies (yes, children are being poisoned with alcohol due to an overconsumption of HFCS). The ethanol produces a

byproduct, acetaldehyde, which is what inhibits the needed methylation and sulfation pathways.

9. **Avoid artificial sweeteners.** They have never been shown to promote health and many studies have indicated that they cause you to seek out more sugar and calories than if you had not consumed them.

10. **Help your child heal from ADD.** Additional reading resources available at the end of the chapter and tips can be found at www.AngelaGriffithsDC.com/HealtheChildren.

11. **In addition to walking, try to exercise every day** (30 minutes is recommended); but exercise does not make up for unhealthy food choices!

12. **If you have a slip up, drink some water and "start fresh"**; don't sabotage the rest of your day just because of your poor choice.

Note: If after 21 days of thoughtfully improving your clean living by following these steps, you are still struggling and without energy, there is a chance that you have undergone a period of extreme stress and your adrenals have been strained or burned out and need help to get reset (think of it as a hard reset on your computer!).

Alternatively, you have had some other imbalance that needs assistance. Feel free to **contact me** through www.AngelaGriffithsDC.com if you are interested in learning more about how functional medicine (looking to the root cause of your health issues rather than just treating symptoms) might help you.

BEST – a matter of scale

Even if you are ready to dive in and strive for the BEST for your health and the health of your family, remember this is a way of life. If you get too crazy and *impose* a way of eating on your family, rather than inviting and bringing them along willingly, you might have a revolt on your hands. If they're not quite there, take a step back to GOOD and work with them there. Bring your kids into the kitchen and start teaching them **WHY** you are making these changes. Maybe even show them parts of this book: involve them in the reasons for the change and they may be more likely to become helpful and encouraging rather than resisting!

Before you jump in here, make sure you have already read through and are doing the GOOD & BETTER lists on a daily basis.

Clean Living, a Way of Life

1. **Reduce the amount of animal sources of protein in your diet (meat, chicken, milk, cheese, eggs and fish).** Think of it as a "complement" to your meal rather than the main dish. Choose grass fed and organic meats, wild when possible, but limit your overall consumption to approximately 10% of your daily caloric intake (maybe even skip days that you consume it) in order to prevent your Insulin-like Growth Factor-1 (IGF-1) from stimulating tumor growth.

2. **Aim for fruits and even vegetables to be a part of every meal.**

3. **Avoid foods you are "sensitive" to** (causes bloating, gas, abdominal pain, headaches, skin rashes, etc.). Food sensitivities create and "feed" inflammation. The most common food sensitivities include gluten, dairy, corn, soy, eggs and peanuts.

4. **Try to avoid foods that mix sugar or processed flour and fat** (e.g. cakes, pies, doughnuts, and cookies). Not only does it spike your blood sugar (which then causes a crash) but it also increases plaque build-up in the arteries. Even when "gluten free," these are still treats rather than staples as they do not build health.

5. Read labels.

WHAT TO LOOK FOR ON LABELS

a) **Avoid GMOs**:

- Buy Organic produce, meat and/or processed foods -- certified organic products cannot intentionally include any GMO ingredients.

- Look for "Non-GMO Project" verified seals.

- Avoid at-risk ingredients including soybeans, canola, cottonseed, corn and sugar from sugar beets.

- By products listed in the Non-GMO Shopping Guide (found at www.NonGMOShoppingGuide.com).

b) **Avoid folic acid**.

c) **Avoid artificial food colorings** (discussed in Section One). Those that are considered same are derived from natural foods (e.g. yellow from carotene or carrots, red from beets, etc.).

d) **Avoid High Fructose Corn Syrup**.

e) **Avoid carrageenan and xanthan gum**. A safe alternative for a thickener is tapioca.

f) **Avoid trans fats. Look for monounsaturated fats (preferred)** over saturated fats.

g) **Avoid products that contain ingredients that aren't natural** – if you can't pronounce it, it probably isn't natural.

6. **Buy local and support local farmers.** Buying food locally means it is generally fresher (the closer from the time it is picked until you consume it means a higher

133

vitamin, mineral, antioxidant and phytonutrient load). You can shop from local farmers markets or join a local Community Supported Agriculture (CSA) farm. You can learn more about both of those options at Local Harvest: www.localharvest.org.

7. **Help each of your family members do an elimination diet (to discover any foods that are creating irritation and inflammation).** Resources for doing an elimination diet can be found at www.AngelaGriffithsDC.com/HealtheChildren.

8. **Help your family detox from chemicals, toxins and "sludge" that builds up in your body.** Resources for detoxing can be found at www.AngelaGriffithsDC.com/HealtheChildren.

9. **Don't have your kids eat school food until/unless you know they have clean options.**

10. **Don't contribute to the problem at school** (e.g. sending sodas, candies or unhealthy food with your child or bringing cakes, sweets or unhealthy foods to the classroom). There are lots of cute and healthy ideas on *Pinterest* for classroom party foods that are healthier options.

11. **Encourage your family to be more active on a daily basis.** Daily walking plus 30-minutes or more of activity. Time spent as a family in activity can improve your relationships, but also instill lifetime fitness habits in your child or children.

12. **Brain repair.** If, after doing the above steps, you still find that you or your child need some assistance with brain repair, some tips are available at www.AngelaGriffithsDC.com/HealtheChildren.

13. **Keep learning about these issues and how to protect your kids.** Additional reading recommendations:

- *The Immune System Recovery Plan*, Susan Blum, M.D.

- *Is This Your Child? Discovering and Treating Unrecognized Allergies in Children and Adults. For Children Who Are Complaining, Cranky, Slow Learners, Aggressive, Hyperactive, Unwell, or Depressed*, Doris Rapp, M.D.

- *Healing the New Childhood Epidemics: Autism, ADHD, Asthma and Allergies*, Kenneth Bock, M.D.

- *Eat to Live*, Joel Fuhrman, M.D.

- *Thrive Foods*, Brendan Brazier

- *Integrative Nutrition*, Joshua Rosenthal

CHAPTER 23

NAVIGATING THE PEER CULTURE

ELEMENTARY: When your child is in elementary school, you still have a large control over their "peer" environment outside of the classroom. But what happens in the classroom consumes six to seven hours of your child's 14-16 hour day! So, 45 to 50% of their time during the week is spent at school.

While there are regulations in many school districts today which prohibit the sale of food items for fundraising purposes, many schools just wait until 15 minutes after the day ends and then sell – and what they sell is generally not healthy food.

There are also regulations that encourage teachers *not* to use food as an incentive or to provide junk food in the classroom. However, I have seen many schools that encourage this on paper but do not enforce it.

Even beyond what schools call and serve as "breakfast," many classrooms have snacks for kids who get low blood sugar or who didn't get a chance to eat breakfast. These are almost always pre-packaged processed foods, which have a long shelf life and are full of Frankenstein-like-food-substances that actually rob your kids of essential vitamins and nutrients.

Lunch can be a mini-lesson in peer-influenced decision making: what's he/she eating, what's cool or uncool to "like," what do others say when/if you bring your own lunch, do your friends *want* what you have (or do they make faces and noises at it), what do the adults encourage you to eat?

Many schools do have recommendations now about how many classroom "parties" may occur in a school year. They pre-arrange which days will be parties for holidays and often they try to consolidate all birthdays for one month into one party (rather than two, three or four per month). But what is served and consumed at these parties is a prescription for a stomach ache and feed into our children's potential development of sugar cravings and chemical toxicity: imagine a Halloween party happening 10-14 times per school year. And they *wonder* why so many kids can't sit still?

I encourage you to start by opening your eyes and simply observing what goes on at your child's campus.

How many of the above-mentioned behaviors are occurring, and how can you start to make a wedge and encourage change? What is the school serving for breakfast and lunch (school-provided menus) and is there anything there that you want your kids to eat? What kind of food can you send in your child's lunch that will make other kids envious or make your child feel like he/she is cool for eating it? How can you find other parents in your child's class that will help you swing the tide to provide and encourage healthy snacks at class parties?

I have seen some absolutely amazing and darling ideas for healthy snacks on friends' blogs and on *Pinterest*. Often times the coolest part is what they are called: Goblin's guts (a green veggie smoothie), Dracula blood (a carrot/beet/orange smoothie) or fruit into sculptures of turkeys, a cornucopia of fruit, and veggies, etc. We really *can* do this!

MIDDLE AND HIGH SCHOOL: Hopefully by this time your teen's food tastes and choices are fairly engrained. The decisions they make when they are out of your sight are a direct result of their ability to logically deduce and make wise choices for themselves (*why* do I want to eat or *not* eat this particular food?).

But there is still an element of fitting in and *doing* what the cool kids are doing. In Section 2, Kelson mentioned Gatorade and energy drinks on campus. Some campuses (not many) still have soda machines as well, but most have been replaced with "sports" drinks. These are all a direct hit of sugar (think blood sugar spike and crash, a set up for insulin resistance, fat storage, metabolic syndrome, etc.). So what can your child carry or consume at school that gives him/her an out? Something to consume that won't be a negative hit to their health. How about a cool metal water bottle (also known as a Klean Kanteen) with either water or Vitamin C water to sip on and refill as needed?

The more your child understands and has a purpose for his/her food choices, the easier it will be to stand up for his/her decisions and to influence others to follow him/her rather than to be swayed the other direction.

This is one area that Kelson has exceled in—he didn't really have a choice. Well, of course he had a choice (as we all do), but to decide to "cheat" meant at least 24-36 hours following of nasal drainage, sneezing, acne, bloating, gassiness ... well, you get the picture. And it pushed his healing back not just days, but sometimes months. He quickly understood the *why* and has since positively affected many of his friends and *their* families.

The ripple effect can be far reaching. Very early on in his food changes, Kelson was asked out to dinner with a friend and his mom. Kelson apologized and said that he had some pretty severe food sensitivities/allergies and didn't want to be a burden on them. The mom eagerly encouraged him and shared that she too had many sensitivities. They ordered much the same way and it modeled to his peer that not only was *his* mom not "weird" for her choices, but that Kelson actually ate the same way. His friend now regularly makes similar food choices.

As Kelson is quite social and unabashed about his need to eat clean, we have many examples. He was invited to a family's annual food fight. Yes, they do eat some and then throw the rest at each other in the confines of a private back yard. While eating the pasta (what else would you use in a food fight, right?), Kelson politely backed off and sipped on his drink. The host witnessed Kelson's restraint and walked over to inquire. Kelson apologized and reassured him that he would eat at home later. The host said, "I really shouldn't be eating this either, so what is it you eat?" Kelson gave him a quick reply of "just simple chicken and veggies" and the host whipped into the kitchen and made them both a chicken breast.

When going out on a date, Kelson does not want to appear finicky or pompous having to ask the waiter: "How is this dish prepared, what is in the sauce, or what can you bring me that is gluten and dairy free?" So, he has learned to call or stop by the restaurant ahead of time and ask about his special needs so that when he returns, he can order simply and concisely with his date. A lot of work? Maybe, but it still allows you to be "cool" and casual among your peers. It's how we've learned to make it work. I would absolutely love to hear how you and your teens make this navigation possible and how in doing so, they influence their peers!

A last and funny example of how sticking to your food choices cannot only be good for your own health, but a great opportunity to allow others to play fun at you, with a potentially broader example to many more. Kelson's larger peer group held a Christmas/holiday gift exchange. Since they generally just exchange candy and such, Kelson politely backed off from participating. A female friend that knew of Kelson's special food needs asked if they could just plan a gift exchange between them. He acquiesced and participated. When he got his gift bag, it contained a large bag of salad mix and a dark chocolate bar. He led the round of laughter, then grabbed and opened the salad bag and started eating the lettuce as is. His friends burst out into glee and then gradually moved about in the direction of their respective classes. Several of the girls walked by and told Kelson, "I really wish more people ate like you do." And, "I really wish I could eat like that." And, "Dude, you make it look so easy."

Oh, it's been anything but easy on Kelson. For all of middle school and his first three years in high school, there has been nothing on campus that he can trust to eat. Our district got a new food services director and we hear some great things are in store for the future, but even the best food services director can't make total change fast enough for Kelson to benefit in his last year. So he will continue with the patterns of survival he has created and hopes that for your teens, positive change is coming.

Our point: choosing to eat healthy, to cut out foods that are contaminated, create allergies or sensitivities, trigger your body to overload on insulin, or are just plain unhealthy, can be difficult, but it does not have to cramp your social style. Kelson stated that, "You just have to roll with it. If they make fun of you, don't respond. They'll learn quickly that they can't get a rise out of you and move on to the next guy." Kids look to pick at and tease anyone or anything that is *different*. Your eating style *will be different*, so expect to attract attention. But our goal is that everyone's eating style will change and you *won't* be different; *you* will be the status quo. But until that happens, find your comfort zone and know why you are doing what you are doing and keep on keepin' on.

If your teen wants support, ideas or just to banter about a circumstance he/she has found themselves in, please contact us through www.AngelaGriffithsDC.com. We would be more than happy to hear your story and offer any advice or guidance that we can.

CHAPTER 24

KID/TEEN FRIENDLY SNACKS AND MEALS

Though it may seem hard to believe, kids can really learn to enjoy all foods when their palates (taste buds) are free from an addiction to sugar. Now, it can take up to a week away from sugar for the taste buds to start to change, but it is well worth it and the meals you prepare don't have to be complex or elaborate.

In fact, while many parents may be great gourmet chefs, I've always kept things pretty simple. The ideas that I will share with you here are basic breakfasts, lunches, snacks, etc. And honestly, you can learn to adapt and make those "favorite recipes" that you already have healthier.

Here are a few favorites in our house:

Chia Pudding
Great for breakfast or a snack.

Preparation Time: 10 minutes (or can be made the night before)
Cooking Time: 0 minutes
Servings: 2

3 Tablespoons of chia seeds (white, black or a mixture of the two)

1 cup liquid of choice (almond milk, coconut milk or coconut water)

1/2 teaspoon vanilla

Optional:

Fresh or frozen fruit of choice
Raw cacao
Sliced nuts (almonds, cashews, walnuts, macadamia nuts or other)
Gluten-free granola

Variation 1: Combine the seeds and liquid in a cup or small bowl and stir. Make sure the seeds are immersed in liquid, not stuck to the sides of the cup/bowl. Next, set in the refrigerator for 10 minutes or cover and leave overnight. Then when you are ready to eat, you can take the time to layer it as a parfait or simply put your chosen fresh fruit, nuts and/or granola on top and enjoy.

Variation 2: Combine the liquid of choice, vanilla (and/or raw cacao) and fresh or frozen fruit of choice in a blender (e.g. banana and blueberries or banana and cacao), blend until smooth. Pour mixture into a small bowl, stir in the chia seeds, make sure they are immersed in the mixture and not stuck to the sides of the bowl. Let sit 10+ minutes or cover and refrigerate and enjoy the next morning.

You really can come up with so many different variations of this simple and highly nutritious pudding. Let your imagination, love for in-season fruits and/or favorite flavor combinations guide you!

Smoothies
Are as versatile as the chia pudding and can be as healthy as a salad.

Preparation Time: 5-10 minutes
Cooking Time: 0 minutes
Servings: 1

1 cup liquid (water, coconut water, coconut milk, almond milk, hemp milk, etc.)

1 Tablespoon flax seeds

1 cup fresh or frozen fruit (e.g. bananas, strawberries, blueberries, raspberries, olalaberries, papaya, or pineapple)

Several handfuls of Kale, Swiss chard and/or Spinach (stems removed from kale or Swiss chard)

Small handful of raw nuts (almonds, cashews, walnuts)

Ice (if no frozen fruit was used or you want it thicker)

Optional: A Scoop of Pea/Rice/Hemp blend of protein powder (e.g. Vega One)

Start with the liquid ingredients in the blender, add nuts (if using), protein powder (if using), greens, flax seeds, your favorite fruit and some ice if the fruit wasn't frozen. Blend until smooth and the consistency you want it. Add a touch more liquid if it's too thick or a little more ice if you want it thicker.

Awesome Oatmeal

*Truly sticks to your ribs, will keep you full until lunch **and** can lower your cholesterol and stabilize blood sugar. **Note**: I always double* the recipe and keep extra in single serving size containers in the fridge. I even enjoy it cold!

Preparation Time: 5 minutes
Cooking Time: 10-15 minutes
Servings: 2

2 ¼ cups water

Dash sea salt

1 cup gluten free rolled oats

1/2 teaspoon cinnamon

1/4 cup goji berries (truly a superfood, but can be hard to find and expensive, can replace with dried cranberries if need be)

1/4 cup chopped walnuts

1 Tablespoon ground flaxseeds

1 Tablespoon Grade B Maple Syrup or Blackstrap molasses (molasses is so healthy, but some people have a hard time with the taste; maybe try ½ and ½)

1 cup almond, hemp or coconut milk

Combine the water and salt in a medium saucepan and turn the heat to high. When the water boils, turn the heat to low, add oatmeal, and cook, stirring, until the water is just absorbed, 5-10 minutes. Turn the heat off. Add the cinnamon, goji berries, walnuts and flaxseeds. Stir, cover the pan, and let set for 5 minutes. Serve with molasses or syrup and milk of choice.

Lumberjack Protein Pancakes

Preparation Time: 5 minutes
Cooking Time: 10 minutes
Servings: 2

1 ripe banana

2 organic, cage-free eggs

1 Tablespoon olive oil

Approximately 1 cup of liquid (almond milk, coconut milk or water)

3/4 cup gluten free pancake mix (we love Pamela's Baking & Pancake Mix)

2 scoops vanilla or plain hemp/pea/rice protein powder

1 cup fresh or frozen blueberries

1/4 cup chopped walnuts

Organic Grade B Maple Syrup

Mash the ripe banana in the bottom of a large mixing bowl. Beat the eggs (on the side of the bowl) and then mix with the banana. Add the olive oil, pancake mix, protein powder and liquid mixing until everything is moist and it is the consistency you want. Add a tad more liquid or pancake mix until it is the consistency that lightly flows off the end of the spoon. Heat up a pan or grill on medium-high heat (I learned it's ready when a drop of water "dances"). Ladle the batter on for the size of the pancakes that you like to serve (we do them big!). Place some blueberries and walnuts in the batter. When the bubbles start to pop clean through, flip the pancakes and allow them to heat another ~2 minutes on the other side. Use remaining blueberries and walnuts to garnish. Serve with organic Grade B Maple Syrup.

Alternative Option: Banana and macadamia nut (instead of blueberries and walnuts).

Chocolate Blueberry Energy Bars

*From **Thrive—The Vegan Nutrition Guide to Optimal Performance in Sports and Life**, by Brendan Brazier; great information in this book also about sprouting grains rather than cooking them (providing additional nutrients).*

Preparation Time: 25 minutes
Cooking Time: 0
Servings: 10

1 cup fresh or soaked dried dates

1/4 cup almonds

1/4 cup blueberries

1/4 cup roasted carob powder or cacao

1/4 cup ground flaxseed

1/4 cup hemp protein

1/4 cup unhulled sesame seeds

1 teaspoon fresh lemon juice

1/2 teaspoon lemon zest

Sea salt to taste

1/2 cup sprouted or cooked buckwheat (optional)

1/2 cup frozen blueberries

In a food processor, process all ingredients except the buckwheat and blueberries until desired texture is reached. If you prefer a uniformly smooth bar, process longer. If you would rather have a bar with more crunch and texture, blend for less time. Remove mixture from processor and put on a clean surface. Knead buckwheat and berries into mixture by hand. There are two ways to shape the bars: you can roll the mixture into small protein balls (storing a few in individual snack size baggies) or shape it into bars. If I shape into bars, I flatten it into a square or rectangle, cut and individually wrap or bag the bars. They can be placed into the freezer and grabbed when needed. They are terrific frozen, or can sit in a backpack or other bag until you are ready to consume them later in the day.

Optional other variety (Apple Cinnamon):

1 small apple, cored

1 cup fresh or soaked dried dates

1/2 cup soaked or cooked quinoa

1/4 cup almonds

1/4 cup ground flaxseed

1/4 cup hemp protein

2 teaspoons cinnamon

1/2 teaspoon nutmeg

Sea salt to taste

Roasted Garlic Hummus

Great to use as a sandwich or wrap "spread" or as a dip for fresh veggies.

Preparation Time: 10 minutes
Cooking Time: 1 hour (can be cooked ahead of the preparation)
Servings: 4-6

1 whole bulb garlic (unpeeled)

1 15-ounce can chickpeas (garbanzo beans), drained and rinsed

2 Tablespoons water or vegetable broth

2 teaspoons olive oil

½ teaspoon salt

3 Tablespoons lemon juice

Heat oven to 350 degrees F. Cut off about ½-inch off the top of the garlic bulb to expose the open cloves. Drizzle with olive oil. Wrap in foil and bake 60 minutes. Let cool about 10 minutes. Squeeze the garlic bulb and all of the perfectly roasted cloves will just ooze out for you. Dump all ingredients into the food processor (or blender) and whiz until a smooth consistency.

Alternative Option: Roasted red pepper instead of roasted garlic.

Black Bean Dip

Kids enjoy dips for everything—chips, veggies, as spreads on wraps and sandwiches. Enjoy!

Preparation Time: 5 minutes
Cooking Time: 0 minutes
Servings: 4-6

1 15-ounce can black beans, drained and rinsed (or 1 ½ cups cooked beans)

1 cup salsa

1 teaspoon ground cumin

Combine all ingredients in a food processor or blender and process until smooth.

Low Fat Guacamole

Allows you to reap the benefit of some good fat without overdoing it on this yummy dip, spread or complement to any meal.

*From **The Cancer Survivor's Guide—Foods that help you fight back!** By Neal Barnard, M.D.*

Preparation Time: 15 minutes
Cooking Time: 0 minutes
Servings: 4-6

1 cup canned, fresh or frozen green peas

1 ripe avocado

1/2 cup salsa

3 Tablespoons freshly squeezed lemon juice

1 garlic clove, minced or pressed

1/2 teaspoon ground cumin

1 green onion, thinly sliced (optional)

1 Tablespoon minced fresh cilantro (optional)

1/4 teaspoon sea salt

1/4 teaspoon ground black pepper

If using canned peas, drain and rinse them well. If using fresh or frozen peas, blanch them in boiling water for 2 minutes to soften; drain well and immediately rinse under cold water to prevent further cooking. Cut the avocado in half lengthwise. Twist to separate the halves. Remove the pit and scoop out the flesh with a spoon. For chunky guacamole, mash the avocado and peas together using a potato masher or fork. For a creamier texture, combine the avocado and peas in a food processor. Add the salsa, lemon juice, garlic, cumin and optional onion and/or cilantro and stir or process until well combined. Season with salt and pepper to taste.

Best served the day it was made. To prevent left-over guacamole from turning brown, cover the surface directly with plastic wrap. Store it in a tightly covered container in the refrigerator for up to 24 hours.

Veggie Wraps

Preparation Time: 10 minutes
Cooking Time: 0 minutes
Servings: 4 meal-size servings or 12 appetizer servings

1 recipe Roast Garlic (or other flavor) Hummus or Black Bean Dip

8 whole wheat or gluten free tortillas

4 carrots, grated

8 lettuce leaves, 1 cup baby spinach, or 1 5-ounce container of sprouts

Optional: Add think sticks of cucumber or red bell pepper before rolling

Shred carrots. Spread hummus or bean spread thinly on 3/4 of the tortilla. Add carrots and lettuce, spinach or sprouts. Roll up each tortilla, secure with evenly spaced toothpicks (e.g. 5), slice into individual rolls if desired. For a meal, cut each tortilla in half.

Guacamole Kale Wrap

Preparation Time: 5 minutes
Cooking Time: 0 minutes
Servings: 1 meal-size serving or 3 appetizer servings

1/2 cup Low-Fat Guacamole or fresh store-bought

1/2 cup black beans (if from a can, drain and rinse; remainder can be reserved for later use)

1 cup soaked or cooked quinoa

2 leaves dinosaur kale

3 Tablespoons vinaigrette

Place the guacamole, beans and quinoa on a leaf of kale. Drizzle salad dressing over the top. Roll up, tucking ends in so that the wrap is secure. Cut into pieces if desired.

Sunflower Seed Pâté Collard Wraps

Preparation Time: 5 minutes
Cooking Time: 0 minutes
Servings: 2 meal-size serving or 6 appetizer servings

2 cloves garlic

2 cups sunflower seeds

1/2 cup walnuts

1/3 cup hemp oil

1/4 cup orange juice

1 teaspoon sea salt

2 leaves collard greens

In a food processor, process all ingredients except the collard wrap together until smooth. (Makes about 2 cups; can keep refrigerated for up to 2 weeks.) Place the sunflower pâté on a collard green. Roll up, tucking the ends in so the wrap is secure. Cut into pieces if desired.

Dark Kale Salad with Avocado

Don't be fooled; even non-kale aficionados will enjoy this salad!

Preparation Time: 15 minutes
Cooking Time: 0 minutes
Servings: 4-6

1 bunch dinosaur or lacinato kale, stems removed and discarded, leaves thinly sliced

3 Tablespoons extra-virgin olive oil

Juice from 1/2 lemon

Pinch of sea salt

1 cup cherry tomatoes, halved

1/2 small red onion, halved and thinly sliced

1 ripe avocado, cut into chunks

1/2 cup raw or toasted pumpkin seeds

In a large bowl, combine kale, olive oil, lemon juice, and a pinch of sea salt. Massage kale with your hands for a few minutes until it begins to soften and turn bright-dark green. Add remaining ingredients and season to taste with sea salt and pepper; toss gently to combine. Serve cold or at room temperature.

Roasted Cauliflower with Cumin, Coriander and Almonds

From Jamie Oliver

Preparation Time: 5 minutes
Cooking Time: 20 minutes
Servings: 4

1 head Cauliflower, outer green leaves removed, broken into florets

Sea Salt

2 Tablespoons Olive Oil

2 teaspoons Cumin Seeds

2 teaspoons Coriander Seeds

1-2 dried Red Chilies

1 handful blanched almonds, smashed

Zest and Juice of 1 Lemon

Preheat oven to 400 degrees F.

Blanch cauliflower in well salted boiling water for a couple of minutes then drain in a colander, allowing it to steam dry (you don't want any water left in your cauliflower or it won't roast properly). Toss it in a good lug of olive oil. Then with a mortar and pestle, bash your spices and chilies with a pinch of salt. Mix them with your almonds and put in a hot, dry ovenproof pan to slowly toast. After a couple minutes, add the cauliflower. When it gets a nice bit of color on it, add the lemon zest and juice and mix around well for about a minute then put the pan into the preheated oven for about 15 minutes to crisp.

Garlic Oregano Yam Oven Fries

*One of my family's all-time favorites; from **Thrive—The Vegan Nutrition Guide to Optimal Performance in Sports and Life,** by Brendan Brazier. We always at least double this recipe!*

Preparation Time: 10 minutes
Cooking Time: 35-45 minutes
Servings: 2

2 medium yams

2 cloves garlic

2 Tablespoons coarsely chopped pumpkin seeds

1 Tablespoon oregano

1 ½ Tablespoons coconut oil

1/2 Tablespoon basil

Sea salt to taste

Preheat oven to 300 degrees F. Cut yams into wedges or chunks. In bowl, combine the garlic, pumpkin seeds, oregano, coconut oil, basil, and sea salt. Add the yams, stirring with your hands to make sure all the pieces are covered with the mixture. Spread yams on a baking tray lightly oiled with coconut oil; bake for about 35 minutes. If you prefer them crispier, leave in oven for an extra 5 to 10 minutes.

Creamy Potato-Leek Soup

Preparation Time: 10 minutes
Cooking Time: 30 minutes

Servings: 4

1 Tablespoon extra-virgin olive oil

2 leeks, white and light green parts washed and sliced into 1/4-inch slices

2 cups chopped yellow onion

1/2 teaspoon sea salt

3 cloves garlic, minced

2 large Yukon Gold potatoes (about 1 pound), peeled and cubed into 1/2–inch

4 cups vegetable stock

2-3 teaspoons fresh rosemary leaves

Heat a 4-quart soup pot over medium heat and add the oil. Add the leeks, onion and sea salt and sauté for about 5 minutes, stirring often, until the onion begins to turn translucent. Add the garlic and stir well. Cook for 1 minute more. Add the potatoes and vegetable stock, cover, and bring to a boil. Reduce heat to a simmer. Cook 20 minutes. Remove the soup from the heat and use an immersion (stick) blender to blend the soup in the pot or ladle the soup into a blender 1 cup at a time. Blend the soup with the fresh rosemary leaves until smooth and free of chunks. Pour smooth soup into a heat-proof bowl and continue until all of the soup has been blended. Transfer the soup back to the original pot and warm over low heat until heated through. Serve hot.

Simple Lentil Soup

Preparation Time: 15 minutes
Cooking Time: 45 minutes

Servings: 4

1 Tablespoon extra-virgin olive oil

6 cloves garlic, minced

2 cups onion, chopped

1 cup carrots, chopped into thin half-moons

1 cup celery, chopped

1 teaspoon basil

1/2 teaspoon thyme

1/2 teaspoon oregano

1/2 teaspoon black pepper

Pinch of sea salt

2 cups dry brown lentils

1 14.5 ounce can diced tomatoes

5 cups of vegetable stock

4 cups water

In a large pot, over medium-high heat, cook onion, carrots and celery in oil until onions are translucent. Stir in garlic and cook another 30 seconds. Stir in spices and salt. Add lentils, tomatoes, stock and water and bring to a boil. Reduce heat and simmer for 40 minutes. Let cool slightly before serving.

Butternut Squash and Bean Soup

From McDougall Newsletter, January 2009
(http://www.drmcdougall.com)

Preparation Time: 15 minutes
Cooking Time: 30 minutes
Servings: 4

1 onion, chopped

5 cups water

4 cups peeled and chopped butternut squash

2 15-ounce cans cannellini beans, drained and rinsed

1 14.5-ounce can chopped tomatoes

1 Tablespoon soy sauce

1 teaspoon basil

4 cups chopped fresh spinach

Freshly ground black pepper to taste

Place the onion in a large pot with 2 cups of the water. Cook, stirring frequently until onion softens. Add the remaining water, the squash, beans, tomatoes, soy sauce and basil. Bring to a boil, reduce heat, cover and simmer for 20 minutes until squash is tender. Add the spinach and cook about 5 minutes longer until spinach has wilted. Season with freshly ground pepper to taste.

Potato and Broccoli Soup

Preparation Time: 15 minutes
Cooking Time: 25 minutes
Servings: 4-5

2 large Yukon Gold potatoes (about 1 pound), peeled and cubed into 1/2–inch

3 cups vegetable broth

2 15-ounce cans white beans, drained and rinsed

1/2 cup nutritional yeast flakes

1 teaspoon onion powder

1/4 teaspoon garlic powder

1 large head of broccoli, washed and cut up into small florets (or 4 cups frozen florets)

Place the potatoes and broth in a large pot. Cook for about 15 minutes or until potatoes are tender (can put a fork easily into them). If you have an immersion (stick) blender, put all other ingredients except the broccoli into the pot and blend until smooth. If you do not, transfer the potatoes and broth into a blender, add all other ingredients and blend until smooth; transfer back to the original pot. Add the broccoli and cook until tender, about 10 minutes.

Warming Minestrone Soup

From Silvia Bianco, MindBodyGreen
(http://www.mindbodygreen.com/)

Preparation Time: 10 minutes
Cooking Time: 50 minutes
Servings: 4

1 sweet onion, medium diced

2 celery stalks, medium diced

3 carrots, medium diced

2 Tablespoons olive oil (or enough to cover the bottom of the pot)

2 cloves garlic, finely chopped

2 cups fresh zucchini, medium diced (about 1 medium or 2 small)

2 cups green beans, cut in 1-inch pieces

1 bell pepper, medium diced

1.75 lbs. fresh tomatoes or 1 28-ounce can crushed tomatoes

4 cups of water

1 15-ounce can cannellini beans

1 15-ounce can chickpeas

1 cup quinoa

2 cups kale, stems removed

1 teaspoon turmeric (or to taste)

Pinch of red pepper flakes

Salt and pepper to taste

Optional:

Garnish with slivered basil or finely chopped rosemary

Place a large stockpot over medium heat and add the onions, carrots and celery. Cook for about 5 minutes or until softened. Add the garlic and a pinch of red pepper flakes and cook for about 1 minute or until garlic begins to color. Add the zucchini and green beans, season with salt and pepper, add the turmeric, stir and cook for about 3 minutes. Add the tomatoes and water, raise heat to high and bring to a boil. Lower the heat to medium/low and allow the soup to gently boil (uncovered) for about 20 minutes. Add the quinoa and cover for 15 minutes. Remove the lid, add the kale and canned beans (add more water if needed), bring back to a gentle boil and cook for another 5 minutes or just until the kale is tender.

Healing Cabbage Soup

Great for when someone is fighting a cold.

Preparation Time: 10 minutes
Cooking Time: 45 minutes
Servings: 6

1/2 onion, chopped

2 cloves garlic, chopped

2 quarts vegetable stock

1 teaspoon salt, or to taste

1/2 teaspoon black pepper, or to taste

1/2 head cabbage, cored and coarsely chopped

1 14.5-ounce can Italian-style stewed tomatoes, drained and diced

In a large stockpot, heat 3 Tablespoons of the vegetable stock over medium heat. Stir in onion and garlic, cook until onion is transparent, about 5 minutes. Stir in remaining vegetable stock, salt and pepper. Bring to a boil, then stir in cabbage. Simmer until cabbage wilts, about 10 minutes. Stir in tomatoes. Return to a boil, then simmer 15 to 30 minutes, stirring often.

Vegan Chili

Preparation Time: 15 minutes
Cooking Time: 45 minutes OR crock pot on low while you're at work!
Servings: 4-6

1 Tablespoon olive oil

1-3 cloves of garlic, minced

2 bell peppers, finely chopped

1 sweet onion, finely chopped

3 carrots, finely chopped

1 Tablespoon cumin

3 Tablespoons chili powder

Pinch sea salt

Pinch cayenne

1 15-ounce can of each black beans, white kidney beans, red kidney beans, drained and rinsed

1 28-ounce can diced tomatoes with juice

2 teaspoons oregano

1 can organic mushrooms, drained

1 Tablespoon unsweetened cocoa powder

2 Tablespoons chia seeds (The *secret* ingredient! It thickens up the sauce)

In a large pot, add the oil and heat over medium. Add garlic, peppers, onion, carrot and sauté until everything is soft, approximately 5 minutes. Add the rest of the ingredients, cover, and cook for about 30-40 minutes on low to medium heat (or put in a crockpot on low while you're at work).

Turmeric Milk (aka Golden Milk)
Great anti-inflammatory drink.

Preparation Time: 5 minutes

Cooking Time: 3 minutes
Servings: 2

2 cups almond milk (homemade or other organic variety)

2 teaspoons ground turmeric

Small pinch of black pepper and grated ginger

1 teaspoon ground cinnamon

1 Tablespoon raw honey

Pour the almond milk into a small saucepan on medium heat. Add the turmeric, pepper, ginger and cinnamon, stirring slowly or use a whisk to gently blend the ingredients. Do not allow the drink to come to a boil. Heat to a comfortable temperature for your taste. Turn off the heat, stir in the honey. You don't want to cook the honey or it will lose its healing properties.

Almond Milk

There are many ways to make this. I warned you, I'm the no fuss girl.

Preparation Time: 5 minutes
Cooking Time: 0 minutes
Servings: 4

4 cups filtered water

1 cup raw almonds

2 Tablespoons organic Grade B Maple Syrup or organic agave (optional)

2 Tablespoons cacao (optional)

Put everything in a high speed blender and let blend on high for about 2 minutes. You can use a nut bag or cheese cloth to strain the "pulp" or just shake well each time you use it. Can be refrigerated for up to 7 days.

I warned you in the start of this chapter that I am a no fuss, quick prep kind of cook. There are so many people out there with wonderful ideas readily available at our finger tips today. A few books that are my go to favorites include:

- *The Cancer Survivor's Guide—Foods that help you fight back!*, Neal Barnard, MD and Jennifer Reilly, RD (I say, **why wait** until you have cancer to eat in a way to prevent it?)

- *Dr. Neal Barnard's Program for Reversing Diabetes*, Neal Barnard, MD

- *Thrive, Thrive Fitness* and *Thrive Foods* all by Brendan Brazier

- *Forks Over Knives—the Cookbook*, Del Sroufe

A few websites that have been very helpful include:

- Healthy snack ideas for kids: http://www.pcrm.org/health/diets/vegdiets/healthy-snacks-for-kids

- Kula Mama, Raising Kids Holistically (breakfast, lunch and dinner recipes) - http://kulamama.com/kula-kitchen/

- Veg Kids & Teens - http://www.vegkitchen.com/kid-friendly-recipes/

- Super Healthy Kids - https://www.facebook.com/superhealthykids

- 100 Days of Real Food - https://www.facebook.com/100daysofrealfood

You will notice that most of these websites contain vegetarian, vegan and or "plant-based" recipes. That's because we all seem to know what to do with meat and most of us struggle with how to get more fruits, veggies, beans or otherwise "plant-based" foods into our and our kids' diets. And, quite frankly, research has shown that the more plant-based foods you eat, the better your overall health. So I'm only going to refer you to foods that have been shown through research, to help your health.

PRIORITY ORDER: Food first, *then* fitness.

They're both important, but you can lose weight through proper food alone. When your cells receive signals that allow them to get all of their needs from fresh whole foods, your skin gets healthy, your brain is clear, you have regular bowel movements (that eliminate used up hormones and stored chemicals/toxins in your body). Then, when you have enough energy from eating the healthy food, you will desire to move more and fitness can then improve your brain health, muscle tone, blood circulation, mitochondrial health and so much more.

Losing weight can be a challenge—it's easier not to put it there in the first place. But it is made increasingly difficult by a lack of consistent and scientifically accurate health-promoting information found in schools, in the public, and as released by the U.S. Department of Agriculture (USDA). Let's start demanding the truth and solutions rather than B.S. and a literal sugar-coating of the problem!

If members of your family are already overweight and or obese, start first with food: real food. Things that are generally fresh and found around the outside of supermarkets, especially those without labels and packaging (e.g. fresh fruits and vegetables) are what you want. Fruits and vegetables are one of the best places to find natural fiber, to help make you feel full, and the only place to find antioxidants and phytonutrients to help your body fight diseases.

CHAPTER 25

AFFECTING SCHOOL AND GOVERNMENT POLICY CHANGE

If you still find enough energy, after changing things at home, to work at changing things at school or even further, read on! Perhaps, after everything you have shared with your kids or teens, they are ready to take it to the next level. Bravo! Who better than to change the world for kids than kids themselves? I absolutely think that they have the ability to be a very strong voice with local school government, and on county, state and even federal levels!

Local School District Level

Start by contacting your local school district's Food Services Director (or similar title) and ask for a meeting. Let the director know that you genuinely want to know what his/her plan has been and what it is for improving nutrition in your district. Some food services directors are dinosaurs who need to move on and you will be working around them rather than with them. My hope is that you have a more progressive food services director who has already been trying to make change and you are just the help they need. Many food services directors face opposition from their staff and many parents. The squeaky wheel *does* get the grease and what they often hear is, "But my child doesn't *like* that" or "You can't get kids to eat healthy food anyway, so don't waste the district's money."

There are districts all over the country that have proven that kids *will* eat healthy food that is offered and it *can* look and taste wonderful. Do you remember "mystery meat" and the warmed up *canned* green beans that we got? No wonder kids don't want to eat it. Yuck! Even for a district, change might be gradual, but without a plan in place, no change will happen. I love that many districts are bringing in organic fruits and vegetables—some for one day each week, some across the board, with local farmers becoming their main suppliers. Yay! Remember, the fresher the fruits and vegetables, the more nutrients they contain.

There are many campaigns and efforts geared to helping improve school lunches (and food in general). You can learn how to partner with one of them to support and encourage positive change with your local district or beyond.

- Healthy School Lunches: www.pcrm.org/health/healthy-school-lunches/
- School Food Fight—changing the way we feed our children: www.chefann.com
- National School Lunch Program: www.fns.usda.gov/nslp/national-school-lunch-program-nslp
- Jamie Oliver's Food Revolution: www.jamiesfoodrevolution.com
- Better School Food Organization: www.betterschoolfood.org
- Healthy meals Resource System: www.healthymeals.nal.usda.gov
- Healthy Schools Campaign: www.healthyschoolscampaign.org
- The Edible Schoolyard Project: www.edibleschoolyard.org
- Alliance for a Healthier Generation: www.healthiergeneration.org
- NY Coalition for Healthy School Food: www.healthyschoolfood.org
- NYC Department of Education's School Food: www.schoolfoodnyc.org

Take away action steps for change at the local school policy level:

- If your local food services director has a plan in place already, ask how you and your child can help.

- If no plan is in place yet, ask how you can help the food services director gather parents together to develop a policy. You are more than welcome to use the information from the first few chapters of this book to help them decide to make a change.

- If your food services director is absolutely unwilling to make a change, go to a school board meeting (they are open to the public) and put your name on the list to be heard (usually there is a list that you have to write your name on when you arrive and you may have to wait until the very end of the meeting to be heard). Present just a summary of each of the first seven chapters about food that is harming our children and is present on school campuses. Ask them how your school district is planning to protect, rather than harm, its students.

County and State Policies

Traditionally food policies have been set by the federal government: U.S. Department of Agriculture (USDA)—what foods are recommended and "encouraged"—and/or the Food and Drug Administration (FDA)—how many toxins are allowed in foods. Also involved, of course, is the Environmental Protection Agency (EPA) as they regulate chemical spraying, allowable exposures to toxic chemicals, etc. However, some states may get stricter, passing their own regulations. For instance, the State of California recently passed a proposition limiting the amount of a chemical called 4-methylimidazole (4-MeI), commonly used for caramel coloring, that can be found in a bottle of soda. I recommend that if you are going to work on policy in this arena, you go straight to the federal level.

Federal Policy Change

There are overarching changes that need to be made in federal policies and there are also specific changes that should be made within various agencies. Here are some examples of larger changes that should happen:

1. **Change food subsidies** (milk, meat, farm, etc.). Congress appropriates money to be spent on food subsidies through the Farm Bill (passed every 5-7 years[xcvii,xcviii]). Presently, subsidies are being spent on foods and substances that are heavily sprayed with pesticides and chemicals and have been shown to cause health problems (e.g. GMO corn, including high fructose corn syrup, GMO soy, GMO cotton, wheat, dairy and feedlot livestock). Zero is spent on organic crops and not enough is used to subsidize, and make more affordable, foods that have actually been shown to promote health and reverse disease.

2. **End *all* food marketing of junk food on television and any media particularly to kids.** Food companies spend millions of dollars to promote unhealthy food in the name of profit. This should not be tolerated, but especially when targeted to our children. We need to protect them from corporate greed!

3. **Eliminate all food that is not health promoting from public institutions, especially those serving children.** Tax-payer dollars should not be spent on the purchase of foods that promote disease. Beyond that, our children should *never* be fed foods that are "questionable" or allow a certain amount of risk. We should only be feeding them the best foods, known to promote health and prevent disease.

4. **Change food labeling to make it intelligent: like a stop light, green (healthy), yellow (eat with caution), red (known to cause disease).** Food labeling is a joke. Do you know that even though trans

169

fats are illegal in the U.S., a trace amount is still allowable? In fact, if a food item contains a trace amount (0.9% or less), *that substance does not even need to be listed on a label.* What ever happened to informed consent? An intelligent food label, such as "green," "yellow" or "red" would allow people to know in an instant if they are feeding themselves or their family a food that might promote disease. Polls show that upwards of 90% of people would not buy foods that contained GMOs if they were labeled. So the biotech industry has spent millions of dollars to defeat any attempts to label GMO food. Bestselling author John Robbins asked the million dollar question, "When is the industry's right to deceive more significant than a consumer's right to know?"

5. **Implement a sugar tax.** I know this is very controversial, but at the very least it could help to pay for consumer education and healthcare (*not* more drug research), since most chronic diseases are related to sugar consumption. We could use that revenue to lower the price of *healthy* food, fresh vegetables, build playgrounds in schools, etc.

With the exception of number one above, Mexico has already begun to implement these policies after they experienced a dramatic rise in obesity and diabetes over the past couple of decades. They immediately saw it was connected to the increased soda consumption and sugar (including high fructose corn syrup). If Mexico can do this, why can't the U.S.?

Suggesting an "alternative" food plate – There are many alternative suggestions being put forth to the USDA for the next version of the *Dietary Guidelines for Americans.* This is one that I am familiar with and believe speaks to the larger point of how the food we put into our mouths is crucial, but not the only thing that affects our overall health. The portions of recommended food types are based on independent clinical research and milk (as just another source of carbohydrates and protein, a questionable one for many people) is removed, and water, an element that none of us could survive without, is put back in its rightful place. Notice, sugar has *no* place on our daily food plate. It needs to remain an occasional "treat" if we are going to change our downward health trend.

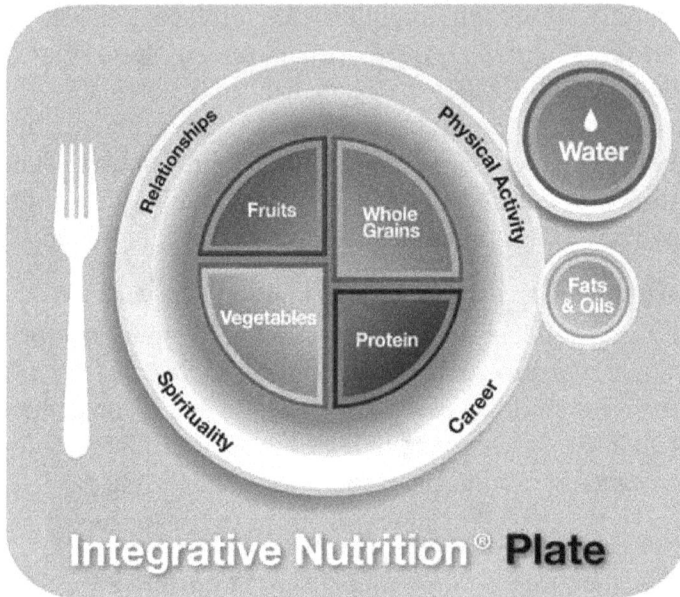

Integrative Nutrition® Plate

Take away action steps for making change at the federal policy level:

- You absolutely have the power to affect federal policy! We should *never* feel powerless. Your voice always needs to be heard. And your voice is heard as thousands of voices. What does that mean? It means that if you fax you're senator or congressman you represent thousands of people by the professionals on "The Hill" (in Washington DC). If you find several friends and you fax several letters you may represent tens of thousands!

- Find out *who* your Congressional and Senate representatives are (if you don't know already).

- Find out what subcommittees your congressional representative sits on – what issues are they interested in? You can ask their staff these questions as well. For instance, if your representative sits on a committee that might be responsible for deciding whether an issue around health, food, pesticides, etc. should be passed and heard by the larger bodies, you need to know this so that you can discuss your concerns with them prior to a hearing.

- Look up their fax number. If you want to send a letter letting your representative know your stance on any particular issue, you should fax a letter rather than email or snail mail. Faxing is more effective.

- Get as many friends as possible to fax letters on the same day. It may have more effect.

- Visit your congressional representative - either on The Hill or in their home offices when they return home. Just call and make an appointment. The appointment is usually around 10 minutes in length, so be prepared with what you want to say. Have your keys points ready. Bring them written out so you will remember what you want to say. It's just a conversation. You don't have to have a speech memorized. Don't stress. Be yourself. You're a parent and you deserve to be heard.

- If your congressional representative is sponsoring legislation that you are in favor of, ask how you and/or your child might be able to assist them in their passing of the legislation. You would be surprised; you might be a great asset to them!

- Attend any town hall meetings in your area. Stand up to the microphone and ask questions. You'll not only be heard but you may find many other parents in the audience who will join the cause.

---

xcvii http://agriculture.house.gov/farmbill
xcviii http://environs.law.ucdavis.edu/issues/31/1/windham.pdf

www.ingramcontent.com/pod-product-compliance
Lightning Source LLC
Chambersburg PA
CBHW060853280326
41934CB00007B/1027